# A Clear & Definite Path
Enlightenment and Health with Yoga and Holistic Living

by Fred Busch

Illustrations by Kwame Nyongo

Published by Magic Valley Publishers
Copyright 2006 © by Fred Busch
All Rights Reserved.

Manufactured in the United States of America

First Edition

**Library of Congress Catologing-in-Publication Data**
Busch, Fred, 1974-
        A clear and definite path : enlightenment and health with yoga and holistic living  /  Fred Busch.
Includes index.
        ISBN 0-9774833-6-3
        1. Heath and Healing. 2. Yoga. 3. Spirituality.
        I. Title.

Both the author and the publisher appreciate hearing from you and learning of your enjoyment of this book and how it has helped you. Publisher can not guarantee that all mail written to the author can be answered, but all will be forwarded.

Illustrations: Kwame Nyongo
Editing: Jeff Metcalfe/ Carlos Portugal
Design: Ruslan Kleytman/ Live Hard Productions™
Cover artwork by Matt Gonzales

To  my teacher Todd Loomis

# Notice

This book is intended as a reference volume only, not as a medical manual. The information given here is designed to help you make informed decisions about your health. It is not intended as a substitute for any treatment that you may have been prescribed by your doctor. If you suspect that you have a medical problem, we urge you to seek competant medical help.

Mention of specific companies, organizations, or authorities in this book does not imply endorsement by the publisher, nor does mention of specific companies, organizations or authorities imply that they endorse this book. Internet addresses and phone numbers were accurate at the time of publication.

# Contents:

# Preface

Many people are confused about how to live a healthier lifestyle. Look around. As a species, we are sick and overweight, depressed and stressed out. One hundred forty million Americans are overweight or obese[1]. Chemotherapy drugs are being advertised on national television. Physical and psychological ailments unique to humans are epidemic. Good health is not normal in today's age. It is time for a different, holistic path and this book provides it.

# Introduction

When I was 23, I was traveling in Africa and contracted a blood parasite. I was misdiagnosed and mistreated and at times, pretty sure I was going to die. Sick and sweaty in a dirty hotel bed, I dreamed about getting healthy. I dreamed about running and feeling strong. I thought about all the cigarettes I smoked and all of the sodas, chips, and fast food I had eaten.

Hospitals and near death add a certain poignancy to your day-to-day thoughts and one afternoon in a Tanzanian public hospital, I thought to myself, 'I don't want to die young! If I get out of this, I'm going to cherish my body. I'll never smoke again; I'll exercise every day; I'm going to be as healthy as possible.'

I did get healthy again and when I returned to life in South Beach, I started fresh. I started doing Yoga several days a week and made some small changes to my diet: no more fast foods or red meat. A few weeks into my new routine, I noticed a difference in the way that I felt physically and emotionally.

At the beginning, Yoga was a struggle. I was far from flexible and most of the poses seemed very foreign to me. I stuck with it and started to become comfortable with a particular Yoga series that moves you from one pose to the next in a way that works every part of the body. As I became more flexible and familiar with the poses I was able to do them deeper. This way, the practice actually got more challenging as I improved. I would feel so pleasantly exhausted I rarely felt the need for other types of exercise. I upped my practice to six days a week and started to become very aware of what foods made me feel good, what foods made me feel bad and what foods made me feel horrible.

A friend of mine told me about a lecture by Dr. Douglas Graham about raw foods. No cooked food? I assure you that I was at least as skeptical of the idea as you are now. Despite my doubts, I sat and listened to the lecture with an open mind and it made sense.

The premise is simple: when you heat something, chemical bonds are broken, molecular changes occur, things are released and destroyed. It is the same when you cook your food.

In its natural state, food has more nutrients, more complete protein structures and more enzymes. When it is cooked, a lot of what you need is destroyed and you are left with something far

*Sick, sweaty and alone in a dirty hotel bed in Africa, I dreamed about getting healthy.*

*Practicing even a small part of the holistic lifestyle you will learn in this book is certain to make a difference in your life.*

less nutritious and in a lot of cases detrimental to your body.

I did not do anything immediately because I was a bit scared but within a few months I tried it. I was not able to go all raw immediately but I began to limit the amount of cooked food I ate and replace it with raw nuts and fruits, especially avocados. A few weeks into the routine and I was shocked at how great I felt. It was unbelievable. My entire disposition changed. Meanwhile, my Yoga practice exploded. I was doing the poses that seemed impossible just weeks ago. I also began to realize a whole realm of mental benefits that rivaled the physical benefits I had already been enjoying.

After several months of practice, during which time I began to vigorously and thoroughly study the nutrition subject, I did not even recognize cooked food as edible. It began to seem illogical to me to eat something with all of the nutrients cooked out of it. Eating an animal seemed absolutely outrageous.

Raw foods and Yoga transformed me. With this holistic lifestyle, I noticed a completely different person waking up every morning. A person who was for the first time, truly healthy: positive, energetic and absolutely delighted with life. That's the way I woke up this morning.

Read this book knowing that whether or not you begin eating more raw foods or start doing Yoga every day, this information will improve your life. Enjoy the pages that follow with a playful, exploratory attitude. If the time comes for you, adopt the practices in this book at a pace that feels right and see how you feel. Practicing even a small part of the holistic lifestyle you will learn in this book is certain to make a difference in your life.

## Chapter 1- A Better Life

I have been convinced that a better life starts by simply getting healthy. We are a species struggling for a healthy lifestyle and in spite of the diets, exercise equipment and self help books, we are still sick, overweight, depressed and stressed out. Normal is not healthy right now. As of March 2004, 129.6 million Americans are overweight or obese. The Federal Government is calling obesity an epidemic.[2]

Yet, there is a clear and definite path to true health. The path is so simple it can be adopted by anyone at any time. Exercise daily and eat right! That is it! I was a double cheeseburger and sausage pizza guy when I began seven years ago so everyone can do it.

We drastically underestimate the importance of health. Our happiness, spirituality, love life, levels of productivity and creativity - everything- is colored by our health. If you want to do anything from regulate your sleep patterns to improve your skin tone, the way to start is to get healthy. If you want to be more attractive, get healthy. Even issues like depression or difficulty concentrating can be alleviated by just getting healthy.

Eating right simply means eating according to your biological design. Eat the foods that humans were designed and have evolved to eat. Whether you acknowledge it or not, every human is a fruit and plant based food eater by nature. A look at the human digestive system relative to that of a true meat eater settles the matter quite decisively. No living organism was meant to cook its food before eating it.

Eating mostly raw foods may sound crazy now but it will not by the end of this book. Cooking your food seems natural now because you are used to it but nothing could be more unnatural. Cooked food offers a fraction of the nutrients raw foods do. In many cases, cooking food actually turns it into something detrimental for your body.

Most health books take an extremely narrow approach to health, focusing on nutrition, exercise or mental wellbeing. Within these categories, many books will narrow their focus even further concentrating on a particular muscle group – like 'abs' - or the value of lowering cholesterol, or losing weight. However, the road to good health requires a comprehensive and holistic approach involving proper exercise, good food and the right state of mind.

*The path to good health requires a comprehensive and holistic approach.*

*You may find yourself capable of things you never thought were in your reach.*

When you start to incorporate the practices of this book into your life, you will start to notice a remarkable change. Your body's systems will begin to function closer to peak performance and you start to feel better not just physically but mentally and emotionally. Empowered with a new sense of joy and well-being, a healthy disposition and mental presence, you will notice your diet and exercise routine take off. They will not be drudgery or something you need to work at but something that comes easily. Such a synergy will occur between your diet, exercise regiment and mental state that you will find yourself capable of things you never thought were in your reach. This is the path to Health and as you begin it, you will realize a new life and a new potential.

# Chapter 2- Physical Exercise

Physical exercise provides the foundation for human health and is inherent to the design of the human body. This is because moving moves things. Like all organisms, our bodies are made up of free flowing systems. Life is literally flowing through us.

Movement is an underlying principle of our digestive, reproductive, cardiovascular and respiratory systems. Keeping all of your systems flowing freely is essential to health. The body is designed with exercise in its genetic plan. That is just how it is.

It is encoded in the design of the body that exercising is essential for moving the lymph and blood and for promoting proper elimination of waste through the intestines and lungs. In order to feel physically well, emotionally balanced and spiritually aligned, we MUST exercise everyday. No animals in nature take days off from moving or from being themselves.

The value of exercise can never be overstated or exaggerated. Daily exercise is the most beneficial and dramatic change you can make in your life. Exercise strengthens your physical body as it balances the mind-body dynamic. This has the result of decreasing nervous tension and calming your mind. Vigorous exercise also causes body cleansing and detoxification due to the increased circulation of the blood through the organs of filtration. Daily exercise is the first and most important step to getting healthier and happier and it is not so hard to pick up.

Why do I say happier? Because if any of the functions of the internal organs like digestion or excretion are impaired, the brain will also be impaired. There is an inseparable relationship between the mind and the body. If there is an imbalance in one, both will suffer. The brain is the organ of the mind. An impaired brain will lean towards depression.

Some Americans lead very sedentary lives and have become sluggish and overweight. Others are forced to overwork certain parts of their body and suffer repetitive stress injuries. Exercise is necessary for everyone, as an overweight person can use a good exercise program to lose weight and bring health to the body, while the person with repetitive stress issues can use exercise to bring the body balance and health.

Virtually any type of physical activity is good for your body, so if you are exercising at all you are off to a great start.

*The exercising is essential for moving the lymph and blood and for promoting proper elimination.*

*Our body improves as we use it intelligently.*

One hour a day is perfect[3] but the bare minimum is 20 minutes and 40 minutes is even better . However, certain exercise practices are infinitely more beneficial than others.  The best exercise is done daily and requires the following: It should involve the entire body, be non-injurious, weight-bearing, fairly vigorous and oxygenate the entire body.

Exercise is best done daily.  It is better to exercise everyday for a less amount of time each session than once or twice a week for longer periods.  Many people think it is the same to practice once a week for three hours vs. six days a week for 30 minutes.  It is much more valuable to practice the 30 minutes and do it everyday!

An exercise regiment must also be non-injurious to your body.  Exercise is for the purpose of getting stronger and healthier and not for hurting ourselves and compromising our tendons, ligaments, and future mobility of the whole of our body.

Assuming it is safe, exercise must also be fairly vigorous. It is the sustained, vigorous workout that exercises the heart  and as it strengthens it, it sends blood through the filter organs more rapidly cleansing and detoxifying it.  Sustained vigorous activity can unburden us of previously un-eliminated waste and toxins. Because poisons are almost fully responsible for disease, lack of energy and degeneration, the multitude of benefits that accrue go far beyond keeping us fit.

Exercise must systematically address the entire body.  Every part of your body needs daily exercise.  Unlike our car and our shoes and a lot of other things in our lives, our body improves as we use it intelligently.  When it is underused, it actually deteriorates.  Bones that are underused now become brittle and can break.  Muscles that are rarely engaged become flaccid, skin sags and systems become blocked.  So the exercise you are doing everyday needs to engage the entire body.  Strong biceps are great, a strong heart and bones to go with them are even better.

Also, any exercise regimen must be weight bearing.  The bones of the skeletal system require exercise to maintain their size, strength, and physiological functions.  If we do not do the correct weight bearing exercises regularly, our bone density will decrease. Many of us perceive our bones as inactive and lifeless but our skeletal system is as alive as any other part of our body and responds to and compensates to the demand that is placed on it.  If we do not do systematic and comprehensive muscular exercises like the sequence of Power Yoga described soon, muscles begin to lose their tone and become flaccid. The law is clear: Nature takes away anything that is not used.

Finally, the exercise program should be based on breathing deeply. Deep breathing through your nose during exercise oxygenates your blood profoundly. The definition of aerobic exercise implies oxygenating your blood and technically does not talk about heart rate. It is said that disease can not exist in an oxygenated environment because they have observed that most disease processes in the body are located in a place that is not well oxygenated. Any program that delivers the above requisites constitutes an excellent exercise regiment.

Hiking in nature, due to the fresh air, deep breathing and sustained heart rate, is particularly rewarding. This is because connection to Nature is often a spiritual experience for people as well. Swimming is also an excellent exercise. Virtually any type of exercise - assuming it is non-injurious- is good for you but the exercise practice to which you will be introduced over the next few pages is great for you. The Fred Busch Power Yoga™ sequences shown (as well as all Yoga classes with competant instruction) are one of the best ways to attain all the critical components of exercise I just described.

*The law is clear: Nature takes away anything that is not used.*

## Chapter 3- Yoga and Power Yoga

Yoga is a vast discipline with many different paths for guiding the practitioner toward enlightenment. Translated literally, Yoga means yoke and refers to, amongst other things, a 'yoking' or union with the divine. There are thousands of different ways one can practice Yoga. Essentially, any work that gets one closer to enlightenment or to the divine can be considered Yoga.

The part of Yoga that deals mostly with the physical body is Hatha Yoga. Hatha Yoga is the form of Yoga with which most people are familiar in the West. It comes from the path of Raja Yoga and includes the Asanas or physical postures, some of which are thousands of years old. On the overall tree of yoga in the world, Hatha yoga is only one small branch. Other branches of Yoga use other means to connect. Many advanced Yogis consider 'Karma' Yoga[4] to be the path that leads to God/Self realization while styles of Yoga like 'Jnana' Yoga[5], look more to the intellect as the means and the path.

Many contemporary Hatha Yogis look to Patanjali's Yoga Sutras and its 'Eight Limb Path' which is found as one of the 'Sutras'.[6] This Sutra sets forth eight limbs or branches which, if practiced, will deliver the practitioner to enlightenment. The original language of the Yoga Sutras is Sanskrit and anyone who has an opportunity to study Sanskrit to any degree should do so. There are many great books and ways to study the Sutras and I recommend their deep study to those on a spiritual path.

The eight Limbs are defined below.

THE EIGHT 'LIMBS'
Yama – ethical disciplines
Niyama – self observation
Asana – postures/ seats
Pranayama – breath cooperation
Pratyahara – sense withdrawal
Dharana - concentration
Dhyana – meditation
Samadhi – state of joy and peace

Samadhi is the eighth limb and in true Yoga is the goal. Samadhi, also known as enlightenment, can be considered either union with the divine or liberation from illusion. However the Yamas are placed as the first limb and are therefore of paramount importance. The Yamas are Non-Harming, Truthfulness in word, Non-Stealing in thought and deed, Moderation in all things, and spiritual Celibacy.

Classically, in Ashtanga Yoga[7], the various 'Asanas', the third limb, were taught simply as a means to allow one to sit in a meditation position comfortably so that the other limbs may be practiced easier and that 'Samadhi' may be realized.

Power Yoga is simply a form of Hatha Yoga. Power Yoga differs from the more traditional style of Hatha Yoga in only a few ways. For one, Power Yoga is very specific about inhaling and exhaling and moving and flowing with your breath. Although this should be true of all Asanas, Power Yoga movements are always and specifically linked to the person's breathing.

Also, Power Yoga keeps the practitioner moving throughout the duration of the practice and delivers the added benefits of a 'cardio' workout. This is special because then it contains all the spiritual and traditional treasures of Yoga and delivers an exercise program that is unmatched.

Finally, Power Yoga is in essence a 'moving meditation'. While you are burning calories, building core strength, increasing blood flow and flexibility, strengthening the circulatory, nervous and skeletal systems, you are also learning to cultivate an inner peace, harmony and compassion that is genuinely profound. The benefits of Yoga are extensive and profound and many would argue that the physical benefits are actually secondary to the mental and spiritual ones.

However we will now increasingly look at the physiological actions and benefits. Each Asana was conceived with close attention to the body and the way it works. Glands, muscles, joints and organs are all targeted in each of the various poses.

When practicing regularly at home, have an experienced teacher look at you every so often to make sure you are not hurting yourself. While practicing Yoga on a regular basis does provide the physical exercise that will help maintain your body in proper

*Power Yoga is simply a form of Hatha Yoga which has its origins in Tantra Yoga.*

balance  if you are doing something slightly misaligned for a long period of time, it can lead to an imbalance.

# Chapter 4- Yoga Asana Instructions

In Power Yoga, there is a specific way of breathing called Ujaya Pranayama. Ujaya breathing is very audible, rythmic, freely flowing and through the nose. Each breath is directed into the back of the throat and then back of the lungs. The transition between the inhale and exhale is smooth and continuous. Try it right now. If you are doing it correctly, Ujaya breathing makes a noise that drowns out the mental chatter. Darth Vader was a master of Ujaya breathing. Imagine his breath. That is what you should sound like.

Visualize that with each inhale, you are breathing deeper than you think you can and that what you think of as the end of the inhale is not actually so and that you can breathe deeper. From the inhales' completion you visualize rounding the transition between the inhale and the exhale. After your loud and thorough exhale, you visualize rounding the transition between exhale and inhale. Keep visualizing the whole time. With each powerful inhale, think of the system being oxygenated, vitalizing the tissues; with each exhale, toxins are released from the body.

This book will equip you with a full sequence of poses that will provide all the exercise you need. Prior to sharing the entire sequence, I want to start by introducing you to the Asanas individually and give the all important details.

**As with all physical exercise, never force or strain and only do these poses if they feel good for you when you do them.** No matter what you are doing with your body, make sure you keep breathing, and breathe through your nose. Keep your jaw relaxed. Keep breathing deep! Rest all the time in the beginning as your body begins the process of getting adapted to this new demand.

Begin slowly and move at your own pace; everyone's body is different. If you feel any sharp pains stop. Use your breath as a tool, both for health and awareness. Your breath has a remarkable way of taming your mind as it draws your focus and senses inward. If strengthening the core of the body, it is fine to feel that it is not easy. Even though your 'abs' may be burning do not show signs of suffering on your face.

The most important things throughout the practice are: that everything with your body feels safe and that your breath is deep and rhythmic. Focusing on your breath will provide many

*Never force or strain and only do these poses if they feel good for you when you do them.*

*Always keep breathing.*

*Please do not do the poses out of order unless you are an expert already.*

*The sequence is designed to give you a thorough warm up to create a safe environment for more complex and deeper poses. Do not to the inversions without warming up!*

*Muscle quality improves over time during a practice. Warming up means that the smaller vessels in the muscles have opened up and are flowing.*

*Warm ups, like the Downward Dog pose (described soon) should always be done before anything else!*

benefits.  If you can breathe loudly and rhythmically you can drown out the voice of your thinking mind. The sound of your breath turns your attention inward and allows you to remain in a focused, meditative state where it is easier to reside in the Now.

The Vinyasa

Technically, Vinyasa is a Sanskrit word that describes placement of poses and their relationship to breathing.  Vinyasa is the way of moving with your breath in a specific sequence.  Whatever the exact Vinyasa, generally while doing the asanas, inhaling is with upward  motions and exhaling is with downward motions.

Always move and breathe completely together so that the top of an action or posture coincides perfectly with the completion of the breath.  If you are going to do a five breath count in a pose, do the five breaths with each inhale being of an expansive quality and each exhale deepening the pose a bit.  On your next inhale, you release the pose and move onward following your breath the whole time.

In the case of Power Yoga, Vinyasa, usually means to go to the top of your push-up, the Plank pose and to exhale and lower yourself down until you either rest  or hover off the ground.  Then inhale into Upward Dog or Cobra and exhale into  'Downward Dog' and  return to a seated position.  However, Vinyasa should be adapted to individual need.  For example, someone with a shoulder injury would choose a different Vinyasa like Core Strength Boat for 5 breaths.  There are many other Vinyasas as well.

The following pages contain the Power Yoga asanas and their descriptions:

*Vinyasa should be adapted to individual need.  For example, someone with a shoulder injury would choose a different Vinyasa like Core Strength Boat for 5 breaths.*

The Asanas:

# Hands and Knees

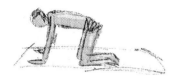

If this is too much on your wrists, lift your palm.

Hands are placed under your shoulders, and are shoulders' width apart, which is a bit wider than you usually think.

Knees are placed under your hips and hips' width apart.

This is the starting point for many poses, including Downward Dog.

*The first rule of Power Yoga is to rest whenever you want!*

# Child's Pose

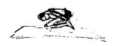

Always return to this pose whenever you want. Build your endurance slowly. Take your time and rest often early in your practice.

This is a comfortable resting position and if it is not comfortable for you, stay in above pose.

This is the most important pose because the first rule of Power Yoga is to rest whenever you want!

Forehead rests to the floor and arms can rest by your sides with palms face up.

## Cow

*Many people have a 'pain between the shoulder-blades'. This sequence is the only way to release that pain because the muscle involved is Rhomboids. Rhomboids is a muscle that, unlike most muscles, does not like massage. However, it shares with all other muscles its aversion to bearing weight when it hurts.*

*This Cat/Cow sequence is the only way to release the Rhomboid.*

*Simply exchange Up and Down Dog for Cat/Cow and watch how fast the knots dissipate.*

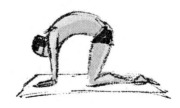

Inhale and drop your belly down as you look up.

Hands are placed under your shoulders. Knees are under your hips, hips' width apart.

## Cat

Exhale and lift your spine as you push your hands into the floor.

Look to your belly as you try to lift your spine 'through your skin'.

# Downward Dog

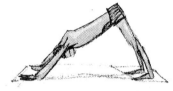

*If your hamstrings are tight you should bend your knees in this pose.* While it seems pretty simple, Down Dog is a critical pose. It is widely used in Hatha Yoga classes to warm students up for the rest of their practice. I like it because it is a gentle pose on the joints of the wrists and back yet, and still challenging because it involves supporting most of your weight with your arms and legs.

From "Hands and Knees", you exhale and enter Down Dog as you turn your toes underneath and lift your hips to the sky.

*This pose is an inversion (it gets your head below your heart). Encountered throughout the sequence, inversions send large amounts of blood to the brain, the Pineal and Pituitary glands. These are the King and Queen of the glands and control all the others. Stimulating these glands with increased blood flow helps them to function properly.*

Spread your fingers as wide as possible to each other and have your middle fingers pointed slightly out, like towards the corners of your mat.

Extend through the arms and legs as you ground the hands and feet into the earth.

Feel that your strong legs, from your feet, are hollowing your belly and lifting your hips from below.

Relax your neck and anytime you want to, shake your head "yes" and "no".

Sense a lifting up from below the navel which hollows the belly. Then feel a grounding down at the base of the thumb and inner heal of both your hands and feet.

Down Dog strengthens the arms and shoulder girdle, general shoulder structure musculature as well as leg and abdominal muscles. Always breathe deep!

Down Dog is a cardio-vascular challenge as it exercises the heart, gets the blood flowing and gently warms you up.

## Upward Plank

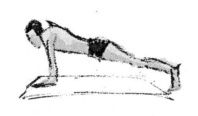

Hands are placed under your shoulders.

Have your hands under your shoulders and then bring your shoulders a bit more forward if that feels good on your wrists.

Turn your hands out a bit.  Make sure the middle fingers do not turn in.
Keep your arms straight.

This is a great pose to just stay for 5 breaths or so anytime you want.

## Lower Plank/ Lie on Belly

*Exhale to lower down to the 'bottom push up position' or simply lie on your belly.*

Keep your elbows in towards your ribs.

Keep your shoulders from dropping past your elbows.

As you lower down, feel that you are slightly lifting your hips and feel the core set of muscles engage.

You must have your shoulders totally over your wrists before you start to lower down.

## Mountain Pose

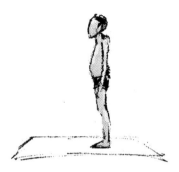

This is called Mountain pose because it represents the foundation and basis of the standing poses.

This is the base pose for all standing Asanas.

Feet can be hips' width or together.

Take your toes off the floor to feel the base of the big toe ground down.

Lift your heart.

*Mountains demonstrate forces of both grounding down and lifting up.*

Let your arms hang down by your sides, lift your heart and tuck your tailbone in at the same time.

Lift the arches of your feet.

Keep a slight tuck of the tail bone in as you lift your heart and take your shoulder blades back and down.

Bring the toes down if you want but keep the arches of the feet lifting.

Strong feet evolve into strong legs as you feel your deepest inner thighs roll inward and tuck the tailbone in, all at the same time!. All of this feels like 'grounding down' below the hips. One Yoga name for this action is 'Moolah Bandha'.

Relax your jaw and begin to breathe deep breaths into the back of your lungs. Visualize the filling of your body with light on the inhale and circulating it on the exhale.

Breathe strong loud Ujaya breaths into the back of your throat.

## Upward Dog/ Cobra

*Always inhale when entering this pose!*

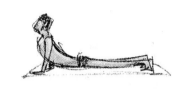

Keep your shoulders back and down and squeeze your shoulder blades together as you lift your chest through your arms.

"Upward Dog" is legs and hips off the ground and "Cobra" is legs on the ground. One is not more advanced than the other. They are both correct.

Gaze upwards.

Make sure that you are protecting against over-compression in your lower back by visualizing a slight tuck of the tailbone in when you are in the pose. Your feet can be pointed back or toes turned under. Feet should be not wider than hips' width.

## Downward Dog with Leg Up

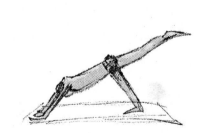

From Down Dog, lift your one leg up off the ground and keep breathing.

The leg can be straight if possible and the deep core muscles are engaged at the upper inner thighs.

Relax your neck. Breathe powerfully.

# Crescent Moon

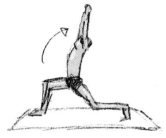

The Inhale is the upward motion.

Back leg should be straight.

Front knee should be DIRECTLY atop the front ankle.

Front knee should never cave inward towards the big toe.

Feel the dynamic of grounding down as you reach up at the same time.

*Keeping your heel pointed up keeps the knee in a nuetral position which is healing and safe.*

# Back Bend Preparation/ Knee Down Crescent Moon

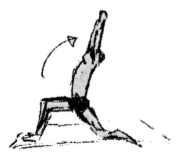

Crescent moon pose with knee down to the floor and back foot pushing into the earth.

Feel that the muscles on the front of the body are beginning to lengthen and open... gently!!!

This is the best back bend preparation because it opens the hip-flexors one side at a time!

Use an extra layer of your mat if you need to protect your back knee-cap.

## Inhale Your Arms Up

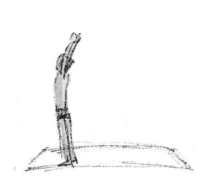

Inhale and raise your arms up towards the sky.

Your breath and the movement are totally joined so that the highest point that you reach up coincides PRECISELY with the maximum edge of you inhalation.

Reach up to the sky but slightly tuck your tailbone in and feel the strength of your legs the entire time.

*A 'moving meditation' begins when you link your breath to your movements. Remember always to just breathe deep and move slowly.*

## Exhale Forward Bend

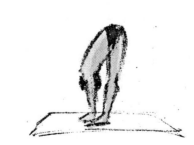

**NEVER IMITATE THIS DIAGRAM IF YOU HAVE ANY SPINAL HISTORY.**

**Bend the knees considerably to avoid straining the sacra-iliac joint in the lower back. (See diagram pg.21)**

The bottom of the movement coincides with the bottom of the exhale. Try to make all your movement align to the breath in this same way!

**Most People Should Bend Knees!!!**

## Side Body Pose

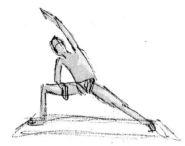

From wide legged stance, one foot turns out and the other foot turns in.

Gaze to your top hand. Once you place your eyes to the hand, attention then goes INSIDE your body, perhaps to your deep breathing.

Always keep the bent knee over the small toe and make sure the knee does not cross the line of the ankle as it bends.

*This pose strengthens the legs and core muscles.*

Front foot points exactly straight ahead and the outside of the back foot reaches to the ground.

As the front knee bends, the other leg stays straight. Then, place your one fore-arm down to your thigh, or your hand to the outside of the foot.

Keep the bent knee pointing over the smallest toe. Do not let the knee cave inward.

Extend the opposite arm powerfully over your head and behind your ear.

This pose lengthhens the Intercostals, muscles located between the ribs, which allows you to breathe deeper.

Open your heart towards the sky.

## Pull on Straight Leg

*This is on the very short list of poses that EVERYONE should do every day. Use a belt if you do not have a 'yoga strap'.*

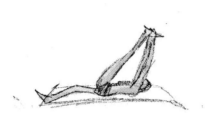

Lie on your back and create a straight leg with a strap or, grab your foot with both hands.

Keep the leg straight or else you are compromising the tendons and not addressing the hamstring muscle itself.

The body usually evolves in a 'three steps forward, two steps back' way. On tight days just observe and do not try to force anything.

Stay and breathe into what you are feeling.

Keep all the muscles of the leg strongly engaged so that the muscles hug tight to the bone.

Do this pose at least 3 times each on both sides.

Do this pose everyday for the rest of your life.

Do not do this or ever straighten your leg, if you are healing a hamstring injury.

If you do not have lower back history and have very flexible hamstrings, you can do seated forward bend if you wish and grab your big toes.

## Forward Bend with Knees Bent for Safety

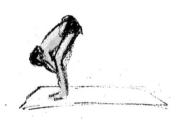

Bend your knees because it releases the pull taking place in the joint that connects your sacrum to hips.

This is very important for all people who want to heal lower back pain or who have herniated disks.

It is almost impossible to heal lower back pain unless you do this variation on standing forward bends. Deeply bend your knees without hesitation!

*This is the most important variation for people with tight hamstrings and all lower back issues!*

So many people suffer from lower back pain and come to a yoga class to alleviate it. If you are one of those people, you must BEND YOUR KNESS AT ALL TIMES when doing forward bending, standing or seated poses.

When I say bend your knees, I MEAN BEND YOUR KNEES A LOT!

Deeply bend your knees, relax your neck and move on to the next pose.

This is a modification for sequences like Sun saluations that incorporate this pose. Someone with lower back/ sacra-iliac pain should never straighten their legs in this pose.

All seated forward bends become exercises in 'lifting your heart' and not hunching over ever. Total consciousness all the time about this with no exceptions and you can lead a pain-free existence.

## Dog Holds Opposite Ankle

**This is an intermediate version that must be approached after some initial strength development only.**

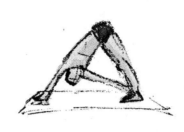

From a Downward Dog walk your feet a little closer towards your hands.

From this short-stance Down Dog, take one hand and reach under and across to grab the outside of the opposite ankle.

If it feels perfect, you can stay there, breathe and eventually look under the armpit.

Always keep breathing steady and deep.

Relax your jaw and your throat!

# Triangle

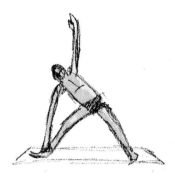

One foot turns out ninety degrees. The other foot turns in forty five degrees.

Keep the legs very straight  but not hyperextended if possible.

Generally, keep your head behind your heart.

Only stay in a pose if you can breathe deeply and rhythmically.

*Whatever makes contact with the ankle, block, or floor grounds down, and the upper hand reaches up.*

*You can always take the front toes off the floor to check into the engagement of your entire leg and core musculature.*

Inhale, reach to the side as much as you can and feel the inner hip crease move deeper in.  Then exhale your hand into position to grab your ankle.  You can hold your ankle (I do this one), use a block or take your hand to the floor, they are all correct as long as you are breathing deeply and rhythmically and feeling gratitude and surrender.  Gaze to your top hand if that feels good for your neck.

# Twisting Triangle

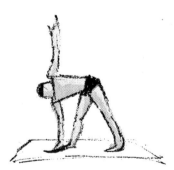

Stance is not as wide as the other standing postures.

One foot turns out ninety degrees and other foot turns in forty five degrees.

Twist and take the  hand to the outside of the foot, to the floor or to a block.

Keep your legs straight and strongly engaged with a scissor of the inner thighs.  Twist your spine from your strong leg base.

*The hand can go to the inside of the foot or to a block.*

*The leg base should have some width so try to keep your feet from walking a tight rope and widen your base a bit.*

## Half-Moon

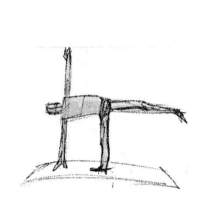

With your one foot turned out ninety degrees, take the fingers to the floor or a block at a diagonal to the outside of the small toe and lift off your back leg.

The fingers are at a location diagonal, both in front and to the outside.

In time, you may start to stack one hip over the other hip.

When the time comes, look up to your top hand.

Finger tips or a block are necessary because a bit of extra height is almost always required. Early in your practice of this pose, just look down to your bottom fingers, it is better for balance.

## Prayer Warrior III

*If you want to extend your arms in front, do so. Keep breathing!*

One leg extends behind you as far as possible. The other leg is standing straight. Stay in prayer position with your hands to your heart.

It is like a T position with your body. Feel the connection of your legs to the core muscles below your navel (bellybutton).

Look straight ahead or down.

Feel that your standing leg is strong.

## Wide Leg Forward Bend Variation

Interlace your fingers behind your back.

Inhale lift your heart. Exhale fold forward taking your arms over your head as far as you comfortably can.

Keep your legs straight and engaged, powerfully lifting from your feet through your engaged thighs, to your lower belly.

Relax your neck.

Breathe Deep.

*It is correct to have palms together and also correct to have them open. The palms together version is a bit deeper.*

## Tree

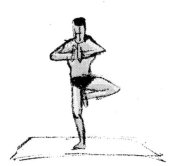

Take your one foot to your inner thigh as high as it goes and do not push your foot into a bent knee.

Keep the standing leg straight.

Keep your eyes steady.

Visualize Roots growing down through your feet stabilizing you.

Breathe deeply and rythmically.

*Take your hands to your heart or over your head.*

## Staff

*Keep your heart lifting and your scapulas (shoulder blades) back and down using the muscles between them and the spine.*

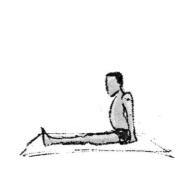

Sit with your legs extended and hands by your sides.

Keep your heart lifting and your shoulder blades back and down.

Toes are flexed to the face and powerfully engaging your legs and upper inner thighs.

The principles of body alignment and the actions used in this pose are to be employed in all of the seated poses.

Lift your heart on the inhale and gently take the tip of the nose down. Keep your shoulders back and down and squeeze your shoulder blades together as you lift your chest through your arms.

## Table

Knees are the hips' width apart.

Hands are behind your back 6 inches with your fingers pointing straight ahead.

Lift your hips up and take your head back.

Fingers can point straight ahead or straight back.

If you are wrist sensitive, skip this pose.

## Standing Split

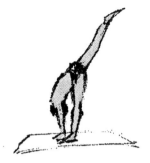

Bring your hands to the floor in a forward bend and take one leg off the ground.

The bottom leg can be straight which lengthens the hamstrings; or bent (with the intention of bringing the nose the the knee), which is sometimes a more intense cardio-vascular work out.

This is the replacement for Down Dog for people healing arms and shoulders.

## Cow Face

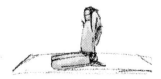

Take your one hand behind your back upwards and take the other hand over top and back.

If you comfortably grab your fingers behind your back and interlace them, do that.

Otherwise, grab a strap and hang it from the top hand down.

Close your eyes. Attention to the point between your eyebrows and breathe.

*If this is too much pressure on your knees, this pose can be done standing.*

## Kidney Energizer

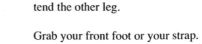

Take one foot to your inner thigh and extend the other leg.

Grab your front foot or your strap.

Lower Back and Sacra-Iliac issue persons should not do the forward bend part.

Breathe deep breaths into your kidney on the side of the bent knee visualizing recharging of the battery.

Feel that you are squaring your hips over the front leg and lift your heart on an inhale. Then, exhale forward bend into the pose.

## Knee Healing Pose (when done with block)

This is the 'knee-healing pose' if you use a big block as described.

Foot points straight back like an arrow and you are not sitting on the back foot.

If you have very sound knees and want to not use a block, it is fine as long as it feels good.

Keep your knees as close together as possible. Grab your foot or a strap.

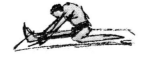

# Spinal Twist

Take your knee up and cross your other arm to hug your knee into your chest and twist in that direction.

Create a twist in your whole spine and neck as you look to the right.

Inhale, lift your heart and the crown of your head, exhale, twist and squeeze.

The leg that is extended remains engaged, strongly flexing the toes to the face.

*Even your eyes are part of the pose, as you look very much right, with soft eyes.*

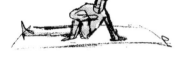

# Fore-Arm Stand Prep

Interlace your fingers and take your palms together with the bottom most small finger tucked into the clasped palms.

Elbows should be shoulder width and should not splay out to the sides.

Head stays off the ground so you are using the strength of your arms.

'Downward Dog' with the rest of your body and walk your feet a bit towards your arms.

.

*This is a great way to build arm strength!*

*Take it slowly and make sure everything feels perfect at all times!*

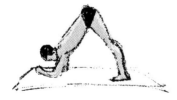

## Hand-Stand

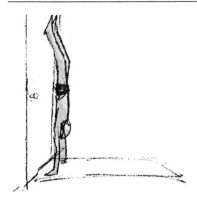

Keep your arms straight the whole time.

Many people can do this pose against the wall, just keep the arms straight!

Keep Breathing

Stay for long periods of time if it feels great.

To master this pose off the wall requires powerul wrists and a very strong core.

Your hands should be like Down Dog- Shoulders' width, with fingers wide spread and middle finger pointed slightly out.

## Wide Leg Plow

*LOOK STRAIGHT UP ONLY AND NEVER TURN YOUR HEAD IN THIS POSE!!!!*

*NO ONE WITH A NECK IN-JURY OR NECK (Cervical Spine) HISTORY SHOULD DO THIS POSE.*

If you are overweight, wait until you lose the weight. Take your time.

From a lying down position with an evenly folded and totally flat blanket under your neck for protection, use momentum to lift your legs up and your hips will follow. See how far down your feet can come to the floor with wide legs.

Always make sure EVERYTHING feels great and keep breathing.

## Core Strength Boat

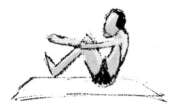

Keeping your knees bent is great, just keep your heart lifting as well.

It is correct if it burns in the deep core muscles below your belly button and in the deep inner thighs.

Do this pose everyday no matter what.

With open hamstrings, you can straighten you legs. In the mean time keep your knees bent.

Core Strength Boat is a pose where, so long as you are not injured in that area, you keep the pose and keep breathing, whether you like it or not. It is one of the only times that it is a good idea to not listen to your body. Getting stronger means that it is going to burn! It is going to burn and you can still be calm. In fact, that is one of the great lessons of this pose that applies directly to your regular life: you can be in a difficult environment physically but still be calm mentally and connected spiritually. One way to know if you are calm is to check out your face for any facial expressions of anguish. Even if it is difficult, relax your face and jaw, and breathe steady.

Core Strength Boat, when done with knees bent and heart lifted, strengthens a muscle called Ilio-Psoas, the deepest core muscle in the body. This muscle literally connects the legs to the hips to the spine and is responsible for your most powerful strength. Thus, if you want to master arm balance poses that are difficult, do more Boat!

More importantly is the way this pose benefits your organs of digestion and elimination. All of your internal organs are stimulated during this pose and in particular, your digestive fire is increased. This is important to maintain the peristaltic action of your intestines to both, cure and prevent constipation. Constipation is very unhealthy. Another very practical benefit is to battle incontinence later in life. Incontinence is an euphemism for the inability to hold the contents of your bladder; it happens when abdominal muscles become too weak to support the bladder and leakage occurs. Obviously, this is something that must be actively avoided.

*This is the most important pose for most people!*

*A very nice variation on this pose is to cross one foot over the other, bend the knees a bit, and SQUEEZE the knees together. Just squeeze the knees, lift your heart, breathe through your nose and relax your face.*

*Core Strength Boat is another very important pose because it develops the core region of your abdominal muscles. It also stimulates the organs of that region and builds strength and fortitude. This pose can help make the difference in mastering many of the strength- based advanced asanas like, handstand, for the intermediate-advanced asana students. Core Boat starts to build your health and your strength from the inside out, the way it should be.*

## Shoulderstand

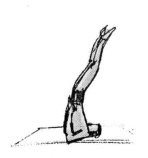

Always use the blanket as described below!

From a lying down position with an evenly
folded, smooth and totally flat blanket that
is big enough for your head, shoulderblades
and elbows, under your neck for protection.

Use momentum to lift your legs up and
your hips will follow.

Keep hands to your lower back.

If you are overweight, wait until you lose the weight. Take your time. Always make
sure EVERYTHING feels great. If anything does not feel PERFECT, ever, slowly
exit the pose.

## Headstand Prep.

**Never attempt full Head-
stand without a qualified
teacher as a guide.**

*Without a qualified teacher
you should do fore-arm
stand prep., and not head-
stand prep. and keep your
head off the ground for
safety.*

*Do not bear any weight into
your neck in Head Stand if
you are overweight.*

*Always
KEEP BREATHING!!!!*

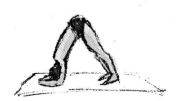

Interlace your fingers and take your palms
together and bottom small finger tucked in.

Elbows should be shoulder width and
should not splay out to the sides.

Head slightly off the ground using the
strength of your arms. Do not put your
head down unless you have a good teacher
to tell you which part of your head should
be on the floor.

Downward Dog with the rest of you body
and you can walk you feet a bit towards
your arms if you like.

# Fish

This pose opens and stimulates Thyroid, Parathyroid and Thymus glands.

Press your elbows into the floor, lift your heart up and take your head all the way back until the very top of your head touches the floor.

Feel your throat open and your Thyroid gland energized.

Breathe Deep breaths into your throat.

*Breathe deep breaths into your throat and stimulate the thyroid gland!*

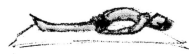

# Bridge

With knees that are hips' width and drawn in towards your waist, lift your hips up and interlace your fingers under your back.

Lift your hips up and tuck your tailbone in a bit.

Roll your shoulderblades toward each-other.

*If this is too much pressure on your knees back out.*

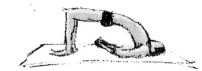

## Corpse Pose/ Savasana

*Savasana is the most important because it allows for your body to restore and rejuvenate after the practice.*

*Savasana should not be overlooked. This is one of the reasons Yoga is so special.*

This is the time for restoration and when you remain totally still, it energizes you.

Lie down with something rolled up under your knees and with your eyes covered.

Palms face up

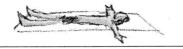

Remain Still. When you are balanced and relaxed and have exhaled a few times with a long sigh, then remain 100% still.

## Crossed Legs Meditation Position

*Sit on a blanket or block under your sitting bones always so that your hips are lifted to the height of your knees. It is important to be relaxed. You can also sit in a chair. While Lotus pose is the most advanced seated meditation posture and the most ideal for bio-energetic and geometrical reasons, healthy knees are much more important.*

Sit in your most comfortable meditation position with your spine as vertical as possible and the knees under hips' level.

Bring your fore-finger and thumb together with the back of your hands to your knees and feel a gentle pulling up from the crown of your head to the sky.

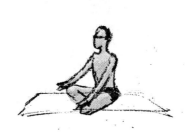

Release the tongue from the roof of your mouth and bring your attention to the point between your eyebrows on the inside wall of your forehead.

Feel that your ears are over your shoulders and your shoulders are over your hips.

## Chapter 5-The FRED BUSCH POWER YOGA™ Sequences

The next few pages will have two great and simple sequences that include some essential standing and seated poses. These are poses I do everyday. The shorter sequence is excellent for getting started. The longer sequence is great if you have the endurance and the time. Chose a sequence that fits in with the amount of time you have available so that you are sure to get in your practice for the day. Always remember that even 'something small' when practiced daily is very beneficial. As you practice, open yourself to feel the sacredness of the 'Divine Intelligence' that is within you and in many ways, is You.

Begin by creating a place that is free from noise (if possible), that is clear and big enough for your mat. Start the practice by feeling the ground and take a deep breath through your nose making sure that it is free and rhythmic. Once you begin your practice, feel a confidence that comes with grounding into the sound of your breath. You become more advanced when you get in tune with your breath. Advancement in Yoga is determined by the connection to your breath and the depth of your surrender, love, and compassion, not whether you can get your leg behind your head.

## Transitions in Power Yoga

There are two ways to transition between standing poses:

Transition Style 1-Change Sides Standing- Generally, returns to a standing neutral position and then changes sides.

Transition Style 2- Change Through Down Dog- Generally, returns to Downward Dog before changing sides.

The following are some examples with specific poses so you can get the idea. Once you understand the options you can chose to transition how you prefer in the sequences that follow later in this chapter.

*Gravity is also a nutrient.[8] We must 'feed' our muscles and bones gravity for their proper development.*

# Transitioning from right side to left side:

## Triangle Pose

Transition Style 1-
From Triangle Pose on the right side, look down at your foot, inhale rise up and simply turn the feet to the left and do the other side by reaching left and then exhaling down to grab your ankle or block.

Transition Style 2-
From Triangle Pose on the right side, simply drop both hands down to the floor and take Downward Dog directly. Step your left foot between your hands, stand up and straighten your legs to set up for Triangle pose, reach left and then exhale down to grab your ankle or block.

## Side Body Pose

Transition Style 1-
From Side Body Pose on the right side, come up and simply turn the feet to the left and do the other side by bending your left knee and bringing your left fore-arm to your left thigh or your left hand to the outside of your left foot. Always do equal amount of breaths for both sides of a Yoga pose unless you have a specific reason to do one side longer than the other.

Transition Style 2-
From Side Body Pose on the right side, simply drop both hands down to the floor and take Downward Dog directly. Step your left foot between your hands, turn your back foot out, bring your left fore-arm directly to your left thigh or hand to the floor, and take your right arm extending over the ear. Breathe smoothly and move with the breath!

The following 2 sequences are of varying lengths.

Advanced students would do a few poses that non-advanced students might not, and might take a few more breaths in each pose but the rest of the sequence would be exactly the same.

These Fred Busch Power Yoga ™ sequences are designed to be comprhensive yet, compact.

## Note:

If you have any injuries or regions of special sensitivity at all, **FIRST** please proceed to Chapter 7- *Healing Sequences for Power Yoga* so you can learn how to adapt the sequences to your individual needs.

Sequence A- approx 20 minutes

Sequence B- approx 40 minutes

*Transitions are Yoga too! There is never a time that we are not doing Yoga! Use awareness and move slowly in and out of poses with your breath.*

## Sequence A

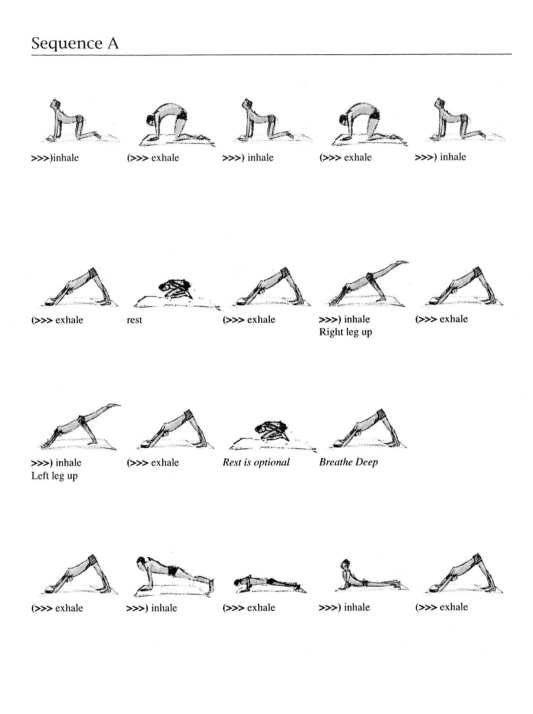

>>>)inhale          (>>> exhale          >>>) inhale          (>>> exhale          >>>) inhale

(>>> exhale          rest          (>>> exhale          >>>) inhale          (>>> exhale
                                                          Right leg up

>>>) inhale          (>>> exhale          *Rest is optional*          *Breathe Deep*
Left leg up

(>>> exhale          >>>) inhale          (>>> exhale          >>>) inhale          (>>> exhale

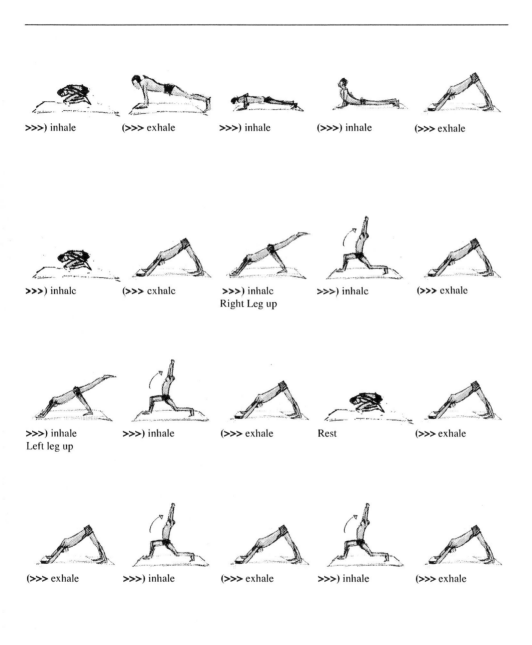

>>>) inhale     (>>> exhale     >>>) inhale     (>>>) inhale     (>>> exhale

>>>) inhalc     (>>> cxhalc     >>>) inhalc     >>>) inhalc     (>>> exhale
Right Leg up

>>>) inhale     >>>) inhale     (>>> exhale     Rest     (>>> exhale
Left leg up

(>>> exhale     >>>) inhale     (>>> exhale     >>>) inhale     (>>> exhale

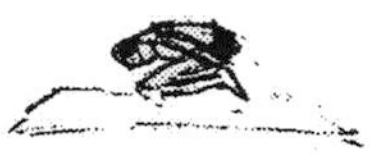

Rest

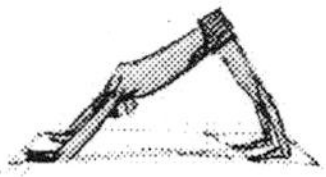

(>>> exhale

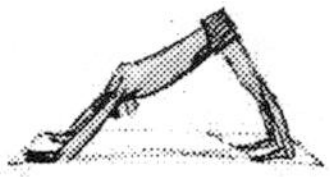

*Breathe Deep*

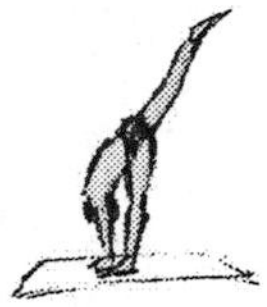

*5 Beath each on both sides.*

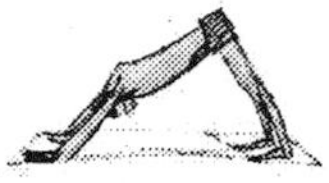

(>>> exhale

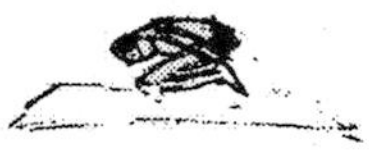

*5 Breaths*

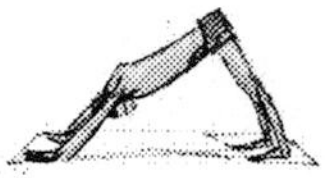

(>>> exhale

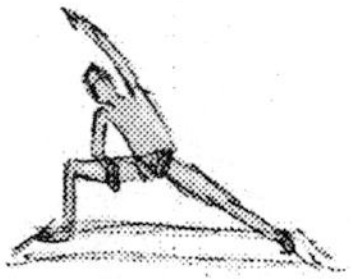

*5 Breaths*
Right Side

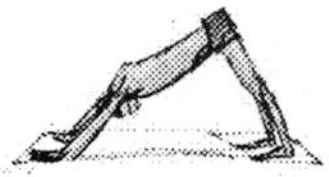

(>>> exhale

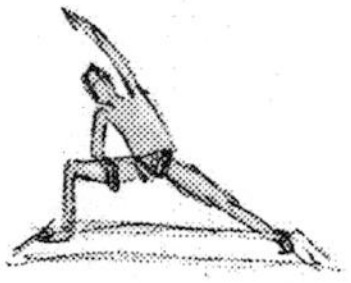

*5 Breaths*
Left Side

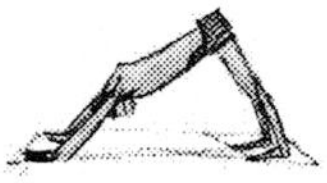

(>>> exhale

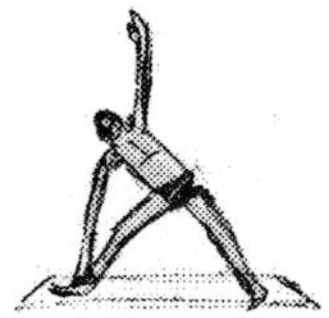

**5 Breaths**
Right Side

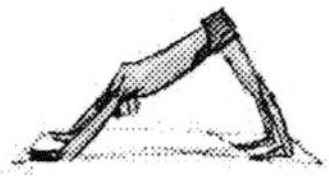

(>>> exhale

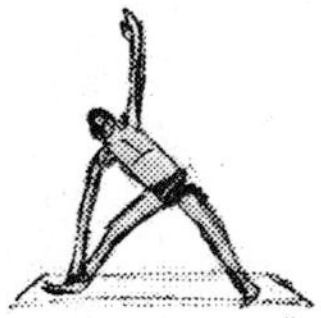

*5 Breaths*
Left Side

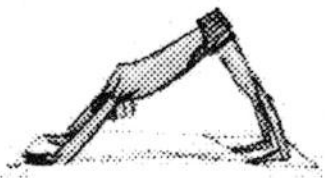

(>>> exhale

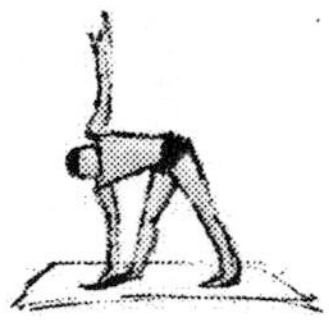

*5 Breaths*
Right Side

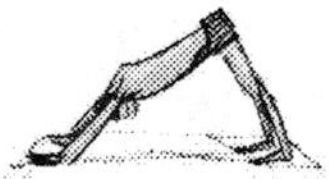

(>>> exhale

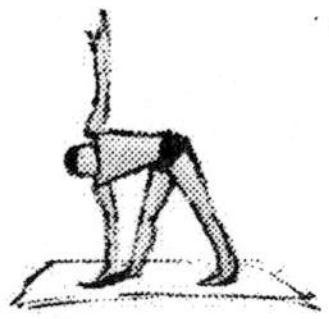

*5 Breaths*
Left Side

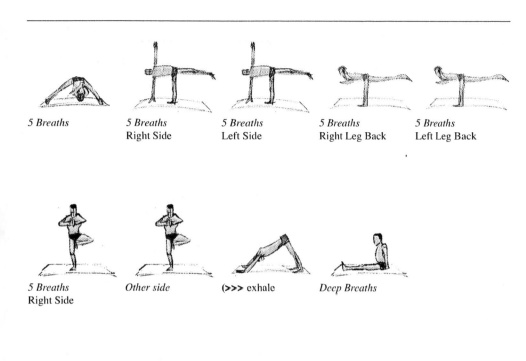

*5 Breaths*

*5 Breaths*
Right Side

*5 Breaths*
Left Side

*5 Breaths*
Right Leg Back

*5 Breaths*
Left Leg Back

*5 Breaths*
Right Side

*Other side*

**(>>>** exhale

*Deep Breaths*

*1 set / 5 Breaths*
Left Side

*1 set / 5 Breaths*
Right Side

*2 set / 5 Breaths*
Left Side

*2set / 5 Breaths*
Right Side

*1 set / 5 Breaths*
Left Side

*1 set / 5 Breaths*
Right Side

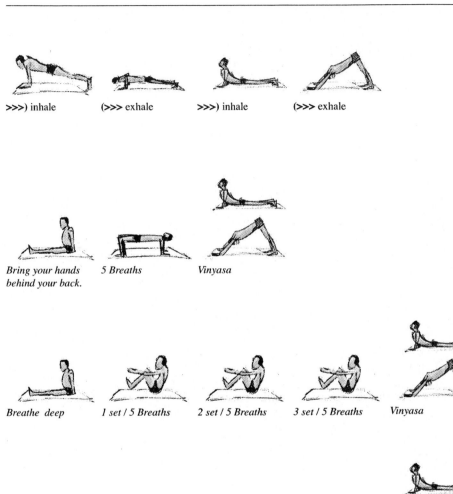

>>>) inhale          (>>> exhale          >>>) inhale          (>>> exhale

*Bring your hands*     *5 Breaths*          *Vinyasa*
*behind your back.*

*Breathe deep*     *1 set / 5 Breaths*     *2 set / 5 Breaths*     *3 set / 5 Breaths*     *Vinyasa*

**5 Breaths**     (>>> exhale and take 5 Breaths - <u>Do Not Turn Head</u>          *Vinyasa*

*5 Breaths*
Left Side

(>>> exhale

*5 Breaths*
Right Side

*Vinyasa*

5-15 Breaths

5-15 *Breaths*

>>>) inhale

5-15 Breaths

*Vinyasa*

*Rest 5-15 Minutes*

## Sequence B

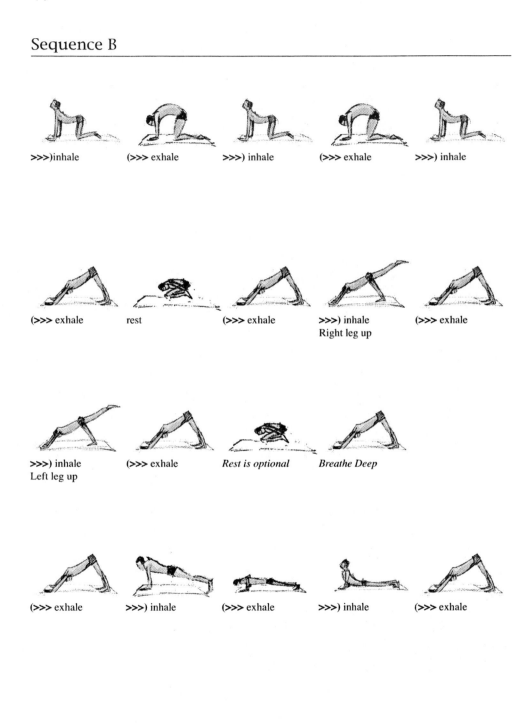

>>>)inhale          (>>> exhale          >>>) inhale          (>>> exhale          >>>) inhale

(>>> exhale          rest          (>>> exhale          >>>) inhale          (>>> exhale
                                                         Right leg up

>>>) inhale          (>>> exhale          *Rest is optional*          *Breathe Deep*
Left leg up

(>>> exhale          >>>) inhale          (>>> exhale          >>>) inhale          (>>> exhale

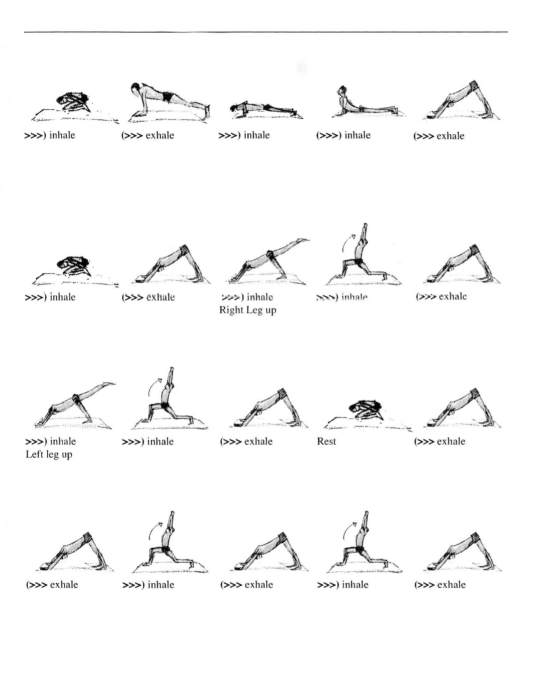

>>>) inhale    (>>> exhale    >>>) inhale    (>>>) inhale    (>>> exhale

>>>) inhale    (>>> exhale    >>>) inhale    >>>) inhale    (>>> exhale
Right Leg up

>>>) inhale    >>>) inhale    (>>> exhale    Rest    (>>> exhale
Left leg up

(>>> exhale    >>>) inhale    (>>> exhale    >>>) inhale    (>>> exhale

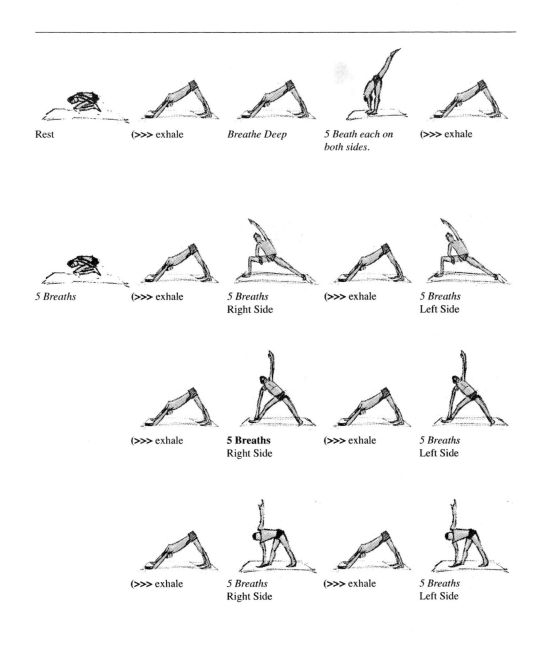

Rest     **(>>> exhale**     *Breathe Deep*     *5 Beath each on both sides.*     **(>>> exhale**

*5 Breaths*     **(>>> exhale**     *5 Breaths* Right Side     **(>>> exhale**     *5 Breaths* Left Side

**(>>> exhale**     **5 Breaths** Right Side     **(>>> exhale**     *5 Breaths* Left Side

**(>>> exhale**     *5 Breaths* Right Side     **(>>> exhale**     *5 Breaths* Left Side

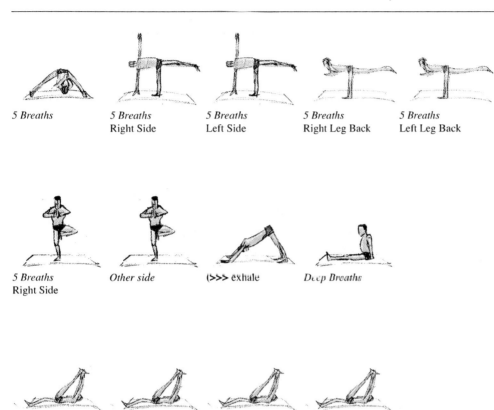

| | | | | |
|---|---|---|---|---|
| *5 Breaths* | *5 Breaths*<br>Right Side | *5 Breaths*<br>Left Side | *5 Breaths*<br>Right Leg Back | *5 Breaths*<br>Left Leg Back |

| | | | |
|---|---|---|---|
| *5 Breaths*<br>Right Side | *Other side* | *(>>> exhale* | *Deep Breaths* |

| | | | |
|---|---|---|---|
| *1 set / 5 Breaths*<br>Left Side | *1 set / 5 Breaths*<br>Right Side | *2 set / 5 Breaths*<br>Left Side | *2set / 5 Breaths*<br>Right Side |

| | | | | |
|---|---|---|---|---|
| *1 set / 5 Breaths*<br>Left Side | *1 set / 5 Breaths*<br>Right Side | *Vinyasa* | *5 Breaths*<br>Right Side | *5 Breaths*<br>Left Side |

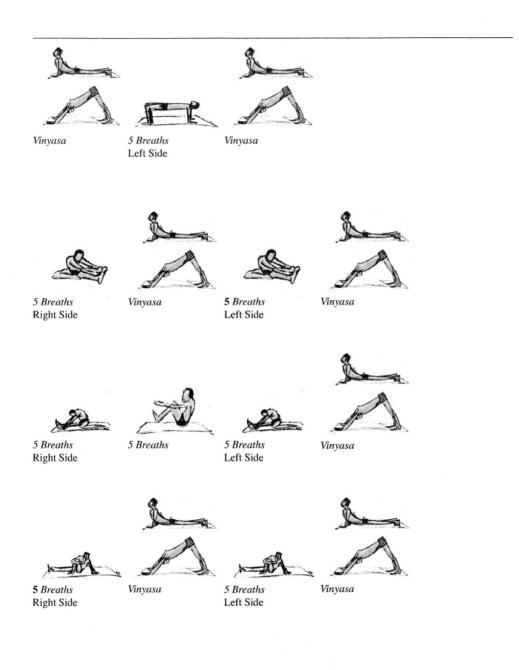

Vinyasa

*5 Breaths*
Left Side

Vinyasa

*5 Breaths*
Right Side

Vinyasa

**5** *Breaths*
Left Side

Vinyasa

*5 Breaths*
Right Side

*5 Breaths*

*5 Breaths*
Left Side

Vinyasa

**5** *Breaths*
Right Side

Vinyasa

*5 Breaths*
Left Side

Vinyasa

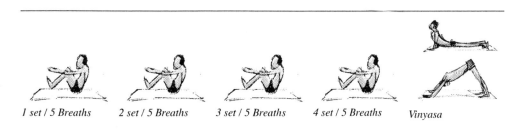

1 set / 5 Breaths   2 set / 5 Breaths   3 set / 5 Breaths   4 set / 5 Breaths   Vinyasa

Breathe Deep   5 Breaths
Right hand grabs
left ankle   Breathe Deep   5 Breaths
Other Side   5 -15 Breaths

5 -15Breaths   5 Breaths
Right Side   Vinyasa   5 Breaths
Left Side

5 Breaths   5 Breaths   5 Breaths

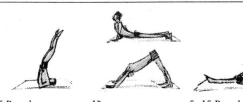

5 Breaths          Vinyasa          5 -15 Breaths
Left Side

Vinyasa

Remain Still

# Chapter 6- Meditation and the Goal

Nothing is more important than daily exercise for overall wellbeing! Power Yoga sequencing brings the benefits of a traditional workout and is being used as the exercise activity on our path.

As mentioned earlier, Yoga is not so much about the physical poses as a real goal. That would be closer to contortionism or gymnastics. The discipline to practice daily is the goal! The ability to come to your Yoga mat everyday is the goal! To live life more fully and with more love in your heart is the goal! Yoga is about enlightenment.

Yoga is different from other physical exercises because enlightenment is the goal. Asanas were created as a tool to make all the muscles and joints of the body healthy and strong so that the body is comfortable to sit still in a Meditation posture. While Asanas, the poses, are just a tool for meditation, meditation is also a tool. Meditation is a method and a tool used for realization and enlightenment.

The goal is enlightenment. Enlightenment is a word for Union with the Divine, Self-Realization or Un-Conditional Love, depending on your appreciation. Enlightenment is through surrender and merging with the Divine aspect within you. Ultimately, the sense of Oneness is with you every moment of your life but until then, the 'Meditation position' is used to practice and once you are fully conscious and enlightened you can chose to meditate formally or not. Most people who have a seated meditation practice cherish it.

There are many ways to meditate and almost all Spiritual traditions use some sort of meditation to bring them closer with the Divine. The connection a person feels with the Divine is the most important relationship that there is. Meditation quiets the mind so that we can feel that connection directly for ourselves. Realized people are connected to the aspect of themselves that is Divine and thus they see first that aspect in Everyone and Everything around them. This is the real Yoga! Stay grounded in the mystical; remember that the mystical is the Science! The deeper we travel in the field of Science, the more spiritual it becomes.

*Yogis recognized a long time ago that with total stillness, a person realizes their own true nature. Once the body is silent and not aching, the person can see the truth as the Divinely merged One-ness that is reality and that God is in every cell of our bodies. And this is science! The Intelligence that directs is in every single living cell.*

"We do not practice to become enlightened; we are
enlightened, so we prac-
tice."-Sage

Yogis have developed many tools for meditation that keep them
from getting too caught up in their minds or from falling asleep
while they are practicing.  One great meditation follows:  This can
be memorized in detail and used every time you take a seated position.

Meditation of Merging
One very powerful meditation technique is to simply visualize
yourself merging with the environment around you.

Visualize your cells are energy and just feel dissolved and just observe the present.  Observe everything that is both physical and
mental without judgment or self-criticism with a relaxed jaw.  The
human brain is very good at wandering in thought which is not
helpful, so Eckhart Tolle's idea of letting go of all thoughts 'mid-
sentence' is a tool that is quite useful.  Eckart Tolle's The Power of
Now may be the most important book you can read if your intention is enlightenment.  If any negative thoughts arise, just let them
go 'mid-sentence' and bring your attention back to something positive like your breath or gratitude. Feel surrendered and empty and
with gratitude and  observe, unattached, the nature of your mind,
as you merge with the present moment.

## Meditation of Light

Visualize a Column of light energy rising from the crown of your head straight up through the atmosphere of the earth and straight up through the Sun to the center of the universe. Keep visualizing that Pilar of light shining up from your crown and on your next inhale draw the light energy down from the center of the universe, down through the Sun, down though the atmosphere and through the crown of your head into your heart.

Now, visualize the same pillar of light energy this time traveling straight down from your pelvic floor into the earth. Visualize this Line of Light going down from the "root" at the base of your spine all the way to the core of the earth. Over 20,000 miles down to the core of the earth this energetic Beam travels and on your next inhale draw heat and a nourishing energy up from the core of the earth into your heart.

Now visualize both energy currents, one from the center of the Universe going down and the other from the core of the Earth going up, MEETING IN YOUR HEART.

Visualize these different energies; one is a HEALING LIGHT from the heavens, the other a NOURISHING HEAT from the earth, both at the same time FILLING AND FEEDING YOUR HEART CENTER.

*While this chapter presents some of the true teachings of Yoga, of which the only goal is enlightenment, the notion that one can skip the exercise and get right to enlightenment is usually false.*

*The body and the mind are not two different things. They are each expressions of the other. If you can not exercise for some reason, enlightenment is still easily available to you but if you are able bodied, exercise is required!*

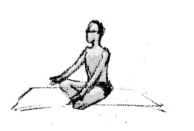

*These healing sequence adaptations are designed specifically to give you the opportunity to exercise vigorously all the other parts of your body while resting the one area that needs absolute rest from weight bearing activity.*

## Chapter 7- Healing Sequences for Power Yoga/Astanga

In most cases the body will heal injuries itself. The body will heal its injuries in the exact same fashion that it heals a cut or a scratch: simply and directly. The only time the body is unable to effectively and completely heal the injury is when we get in the way. We get in the way by using the muscles in a weight bearing way and thereby aggravate the situation.

A muscle spasm is a contraction that has been ordered by the brain so the region inside the contraction will not be disturbed as 'repairs' are made to it. When the repairs have been made, the brain signals the muscle to release. The muscle will not release in a permanent way without the order from the brain after it has determined the injury healed.

Many people stretch into a tight area to try to open it up but usually this is just stretching a muscle that is trying to stay closed for a reason and healing is thwarted.

These healing sequence adaptations are designed specifically to give you the opportunity to exercise vigorously all the other parts of your body while resting the one area that needs absolute rest from weight bearing activity.

I try to avoid injuries at all costs but they may happen. Look at Injuries as a type of opportunity. Take good care of them early by not aggravating the area until it feels perfect. Do not let them stop your practice. They will give you a chance to focus on different parts of your practice and maybe try some new poses. Heal quickly and enjoy the process. Taking days off exercise will never help heal anything, but you must take days off the area that needs the rest. There are plenty of solid poses you can do instead to give certain areas of your body a break when they need it. Here are my favorites:

*The best way to avoid all injury is to move slowly into and out of every pose and to listen to your body. If you feel anything that is not perfect back out and reassess if that action is wise for you in that moment. The body tries to warn us BEFORE an injury happens that something unwise is taking place. Listen and keep breathing.*

# Lower Back/ Sacra-Iliac/ Herniated Disc issues

These adjutments involve always bending your knees in forward bends. They are designed for people who have pain in their lower back and in particular the sacra-iliac joint which is where the sacrum joins the hip, and issues of herniated disks. Sacra-iliac pain is usually felt on one side or the other and is near the top corner of the triangular shaped sacrum in your low back above your buttocks. The sacrum is a big bone so the triangle that it creates fills up a sizable section of the region behind the hips.

If your lower back pain is in a different location, this is still a wise course of action. Herniated discs need to be approached with unbelievable caution. Never let a teacher push you down in forward bend if you have a herniated disk. In fact everone with tight hamstrings who wants to PREVENT injuries in the lower back should usually avoid staight leg forward bends.

In general, teachers should not be pushing their students down in forward bends because it creates a 'tug of war' between the tight hamstrings and the vulnerable sacral and spinal ligaments.

Avoid all standing forward bends with straight legs except for 'Wide Leg' Forward Bends. Forward Bends without wide legs must have bent knees to protect the lower back and allow it to heal.

Avoid all seated forward bending that rounds your back and stresses the sacra-iliac joint, the joint that connects your sacrum to your ileum located at the lower back just above the buttocks.

Make sure you practice the 'Lie on Back and Pull on Straight Leg Pose' everyday. This is the way you can lengthen your hamstrings systematically without injuring or re-aggravating your lower back or sacra-iliac joint.

## Injured/Sore Wrists

Never let your wrist flex past the angle it is in when in Downward Dog.

Avoid Upward Dog.

Avoid Plank Poses.

Only do Downward Dog.

Upward Dog and Plank poses place the wrist at a demanding angle that aggravates the wrists and thus prevents healing.

Stay in Down Dog for the whole warm up sequence and move into and out of the Downward Dog with Leg Up.

In order to really get the wrist to feel better you can not do Upward Dog, or the Plank poses even once! That is the point-no exceptions when you want to heal. Always do Down Dog, never do Upward Dog. If you want a 'Back Bend' pose, you can do 'Cobra' with your fore-arms to the floor instead of your hands.

One thing that many people who practice 'asana' do not appreciate is that all it takes is ONCE to do an unintillegent action and the injury is re-aggravated. Once an injury has been re-aggravated, or made worse, it is like starting all over again. Injuries and situations take a bit of time, nothing can happen overnight, but the fact that it feels a bit better every day should tell you that you have begun the process of healing and in short order it will probably feel all better. Once it does feel better, DO NOT GO BACK to the avoided poses for an additional two weeks to allow for the body's real 'finish work' to take place.

# Knees

Do not ever aggravate your knee for the sake of a yoga pose. Avoid all half and full Lotus variations. Take great care of your knees and they will heal.

Avoid all seated poses which make it feel like there is a pressure on your knee that is not the 'same on both sides.'

Also avoid Kidney Energizer pose if you feel sensations in your knee.

Always replace any pose you do not feel perfect in with Knee Healing pose. Use a block EVERY TIME under the opposite hip!

Lotus pose does not signify an advanced yoga practice if it injures your knees as you are doing it.. That is a form of violence.

If doing a classical version of Warrior 1 in your practice, do not turn that back heal 'out' and instead keep it pointing up.

# Arms or Shoulders

With essentially no exceptions, try not to bear weight into the injured joint. Injured joints contain muscles that are in 'compensation mode' and need to be left alone so they can enjoy the blood flow from the exercise but not get aggravated enduring any kind of weight bearing demand.

Replace Downward Dog, Upward Dog and the Plank Poses with Standing Splits.

If possible, do Power Yoga everyday so you heal but under no circumstances bear body weight into the arm or shoulder.

Standing Split is a nice alternative to Downward Dog because it is a demanding, inverted pose that can function as a warm up without putting weight on the arms.

# Section II
## A Natural Diet is Nature's Will

*Holistic eating means eating natural foods.*

## Chapter 8- Thriving

*Human resilience is most formidable.*

People take their bodies for granted. We know that certain foods are bad for us but we eat them anyway. 'It won't kill us,' we reason and decide to go ahead and indulge. Biological resilience is demonstrated by millions of people who injure themselves with a poor diet year after year and still manage to survive. Like all living organisms we are endowed with a spectacular resilience. This resilience and versatility of the human body has caused many people to become accustomed to treating their bodies like garbage disposers, capable of taking in a broad range of food items and living in spite of it.

However, there is an important distinction to be made between surviving and thriving. The body can exist on various levels of health, without really being healthy. Low quality foods let you live but keep you from thriving. All organisms can live in a range of conditions, but the conditions that are ideal for them are pretty well defined. The conditions in which they thrive are specific.

Contrary to our 'it won't kill us' mentality, consumption of poor quality food is killing us. Slowly. It is contributing to a system of cause and effect that takes us further and further away from true health and prevents us from thriving. The combination of one dietary disaster after another results in a gradual erosion of our health that we may not feel the moment we are chewing the doughnut. Instead, the effects compound and manifest themselves further down the road in the form of some serious ailment.

By slowly and incrementally distancing ourselves from our optimum physical and mental conditions, we become familiar with each phase of compromised health along the way. Since this erosion of our true health and potential is realized so gradually, it somehow becomes acceptable to people. With the information presented in this book and self-observation, you can realize the optimal conditions for yourself as an organism. Once you identify them, which you will fairly easily, you will be able to make healthy decisions and adopt a healthy lifestyle if you wish and see for yourself what it feels like to thrive.

One common reaction to this understanding is 'Yeah, but, we have been eating cooked food for years.' Yeah we have. And we are all kind of messed up. We are all plagued by a bunch of mysterious diseases like diabetes and cancer that attack exclusively humans.  No argument that hinges on humans being healthy as a species is very sound.  Given our current state,  because we have been it doing for years, is probably reason to stop doing it.

*No argument that hinges on humans being healthy as a species is very sound.*

## Chapter 9- A Natural Diet

*Do not be concerned with being on a diet ever again.*

Before you waste any time thinking about what food is good for you and what food is bad, start with the question of what is food? Our definition of food has expanded to include all sorts of things that are not nourishing, that are not natural and actually harm your body.

The only things I consider food are those that nourish my body without causing it any harm. You can put whatever you want into your mouth but only the things that are nourishing you without any adverse effects are the things you should think of as food. Once you do that, eating properly is easy. There is no dieting involved. This is far from a raw foods diet. This is simply understanding how your body works and then acting accordingly.

For all living organisms there are two categories: foods that nourish a body and foods that hurt it. Would a zoo curator feed the chimpanzees some bad food along with some good food? Or perhaps a range of foods, some high quality, some lower quality and on occasion, some down right junk food?

Should we not treat our bodies with the same respect and concern that we demonstrate toward our cars or the monkeys in the zoo? We do not feed the Chimps deep-dish pizza. The vet's job is to keep the animal in perfect health and it is scientific fact that this is done by strict adherence to the animal's natural diet. Your body is designed (or evolved) to assimilate its nutrients from specific sources. Compromises in those sources lead to compromises in your body's functioning and ultimately, your life's quality. You are a human; eat like one.

Once food has been defined, there is no need to be on a diet. You can eat as much food as you want. There is no need to count calories or earn 'food points'; no need to get involved with the latest theories about eating all protein or all carbohydrates. Now you can relax because once you are eating food, you can eat as much as you want. Release yourself from the diet mentality and out of the deprivation psychology that goes along with it.

Do not be concerned with being on a diet ever again. Just eat the things that are food. You can eat as many bananas as you want, you can eat as many apples as you want, you can eat as much raw almond butter as you want. As long as you are exercising everyday it is only going to make you healthier and bring you towards your natural bodyweight.

One way to help you define what is food and what is not is to keep in mind that everything that goes into our mouths becomes our blood. The quality of our blood is impacted directly by what we eat. How long it takes a cut to heal is a function of the quality of your blood which in turn is a function of what you are eating -That makes sense right? So things that make clean healthy blood are the things that are food. You can call all the other stuff whatever you want and you can even eat it if you wish, just do not think of it as food.

*How long it takes something to heal is a function of the quality of your blood.*

## Chapter 10- Holistic Raw Foods

You are literally made out of the food you eat. There is no way around that. This is incredibly basic, but it is something you may not think about. Think about it. Do you want to be an apple? Or do you want to be a glazed doughnut?

The processes going on inside you right now are intricate and precise. Living tissue is being constructed. Neurotransmitters are sending and receiving billions of messages every minute. Enzymes and co-enzymes (vitamins) are working as catalysts; minerals and amino acids are being used as building blocks.

For humans eating more raw plant food like fruits is a natural choice, literally. We clearly exist within the body of a primate. The difference in intelligence between the different primate species does not affect the digestive anatomy a bit. As Homo sapiens, we humans have the same digestive structures as the other big brained fruit eating primates. It is interesting to note that one could easily produce cancer or heart disease or any number of disease processes in other primate species if we supplied them with the food that we ourselves eat.

When you eat cooked food, you deprive your body of the things it needs and subject it to things it does not need. In its raw, natural state, each whole food contains a nutritional package complete with essential vitamins, amino acids, minerals and enzymes. Enzymes are the compounds our bodies use to drive the various millions of chemical reactions responsible for everything from digestion to the production and transmission of hormones.

Think back to your high school chemistry days and how you learned that when you heat a molecule, you change its chemical structure. Chemical bonds are broken, electrons are lost and with them the cell's integrity. Completely new compounds are also created. The same thing is happening when you heat the molecules that make up your food. At temperatures above 120°F, essential compounds are drastically changed and in many cases destroyed.

Water-soluble vitamins, such as the entire family of the Vitamin B complex, are some of the first to go[9]. Enzymes suffer the same fate during the cooking process. Proteins can be destroyed entirely or become coagulated to a point where they are completely useless to the body. Heat, chemically changes food and it is not for the better.

It does not matter whether you eat all raw foods or not. Any amount that you improve your food selections, even the smallest amount, is a positive and significant event. Every time you grab an apple instead of a candy bar it is profound. The best food selections come from the raw plant kingdom but the goal is to do your best and take it slow. Remember that we are not judging good or bad; right or wrong here. Even the smallest positive change is huge. Many people think it is not worth it to do something small so they never do anything at all. Do something small, it makes a big difference!

As will be addressed in a bit more detail later, the most important thing to anybody's food selection 'evolution' is to never cast judgment or direct criticism toward yourself. We can achieve change through awareness, compassion and non-judgment toward ourselves. This creates the environment for increased strength reserves and thus **power** so that you can act whenever you feel ready.

*It does not matter whether you eat all raw foods or not. Every time you grab an apple instead of a candy bar it is profound.*

# Benefits of more holistic Raw Foods

<u>Weight Issues</u>- Being overweight wreaks havoc on your body. Even a few extra pounds creates a stress on your body. When you start eating RAW, if you are overweight you will lose weight! If you are underweight, you will gain weight! Weight problems are unheard of among other organisms (save those that have been domesticated by humans). Have you ever seen an overweight tiger lumbering through the jungle? When you start eating natural raw foods, maintaining your natural body weight will no longer be a battle. There will be no need to count any calories and nothing to feel guilty about. Maintaining a natural diet will come **naturally**.

<u>Mental Acuity</u>- Believe it or not, eating RAW will improve your attitude and enable you to be more focused. What we regard as thoughts are transferred from one neuron to another in a language of electrical communication. The electricity and the nerves that carry the signals are created directly from the foods you eat. With better foods, you experience increased mental capacity and the ability to think more clearly.

<u>Energy Levels</u>- When your body is burdened under toxins, it is hard to pursue life with much vigor. Once you are freed from the burden of what you used to eat, you will find that your body has more energy available for other things. Energy that you can feel will increase, as will the more important and deeper energy stores that start the cleansing processes of the body.

<u>Strength</u>- The first step to being a body builder is eating foods that build bodies. When you are eating RAW foods, your tissues are being constructed with only high quality material and you will feel the difference.

<u>Your bowels will begin to function regularly</u>- Most people do not want to talk about it but constipation is a very common problem. Our intestines have great difficulty dealing with toxic substances and as a result, our digestive system breaks down. Eating natural foods means digestive and eliminatory organs function more optimally. This benefit alone is worth a lot because constipation is the root of most diseases.

Overall Health- There no longer is any questioning that there is a direct correlation between a bad diet and the development of disease including cancer and heart disease.

Beauty!- This is a no-brainer. High quality, clean food leads to bright eyes, healthy skin and toned muscles. Also, happy people are always better looking. When you are no longer going through life constipated and poisoned, it will be much easier to keep a pleasant disposition. Being healthy and looking good are the same.

Helps Depression- There is a direct correlation between the food you eat and the way that your brain works. Long before your skin breaks out or your clothes get tight from eating improper foods, your thoughts are affected. The brain is the most complex organ of all and is subsequently the most sensitive. It requires a perfect blood ph and blood sugar level. Negativity, nervousness, depression, fatigue; these are serious symptoms and could be things that require the help of a professional. More than likely though, they result from eating poor food. The overlooked connection between brain functioning and food intake should be exposed once and for all. Those who consider depression to be a disease or coincidence may be correct but they all too quickly prescribe powerful toxic chemicals to alleviate nutritional imbalance symptoms. Let's have a look instead at the more logical, root of the problem.

*Alleviate depression by eating better! You may be surprised what nourishing your body could do for your brain.*

## Chapter 11- Meat

*Cooked meat is not even good for carnivores!*

Our bodies are not designed to eat animals. Undeniable differences between the digestive system of a primate and a carnivore make the point rather decisively. A meat eater's digestive system is short, efficient and direct. The food that it eats does not linger in its stomach or intestines for very long.

Like other great apes, our digestive system involves a long network of intestines that is roughly twelve times the length of our bodies. It makes a series of intricate twists and turns and has many convolutions for bits of meat to get lodged in and rot[10]. Due to the incompatibility between flesh and our intestinal tract, when humans eat meat and animal products, these substances may get stuck and sit in the stomach and intestines for days. It is safe to say that having putrefying substances, especially flesh, sitting stagnant in your digestive track is not ideal.

Often, I hear people suggest that meat is a source of superior protein as the justification for eating animal flesh. The commonly held superior protein status of meat is what Dr. Robert Snaidach calls a 'colossal error'. For one, the body does not use protein in the form that it is eaten, and second, meat has too many undesirable attributes to make it superior to anything. Our bodies do not use proteins in the form in which we eat them. If we eat animals to get protein, our bodies are forced to deconstruct the animal's protein into amino acids. Only amino acids are useful because that is what our body uses to construct its own cells, its own proteins.

Animal protein MUST be deconstructed to the amino acid level before human protein construction can occur. Our body combines these amino acids to construct its own human proteins from scratch. So the only thing necessary to obtain is the correct distribution of all necessary amino acids. Nothing else is required except that these amino acids must be consumed raw to be of value. Any builder knows not to torch the materials before construction begins.

Because the meat equals protein and muscles mentality has become so entrenched in our society, it may be difficult at first to accept that raw food is a more desirable source of protein. But for primates, the highest quality amino acids do not come from cooked meat. Cooked meat is not even good for carnivores![11] This is because when protein is cooked, most of the essential amino acids are damaged or destroyed.

Every human is a vegetarian (frugivore) whether they like it or not. Whether they decide to eat flesh or not, they are still primates according to their digestive design. Consider what other mammals are eating. Each species eats according to its design. A gazelle eats almost exclusively grass. Carnivores in nature eat their animal whole and raw including the blood and organ meat. Primates mainly eat fruit and plant based foods. Omnivores like pigs and rats eat everything.

Herbivores eat only fresh grass and their entire body structure gets built. The biggest mammals on the planet have been the herbivores, the grass eaters! All proteins of those enormous herbivores' bodies are synthesized from the proteins derived from the grass. I want you to picture that the reason why it is nutritious for a carnivore to eat an herbivore is because a real carnivore eats the entirety of the body and brain of the animal it has just killed and does so in order to get the nutritional value inherent in the grass.

Plants can take the lifeless materials of the air, water and soil, combine them with the photons of the sun and raise them to the status of a living structure. The living structure that the plant produces is called a Carbohydrate[12]. The Cycle of Life starts with the sun's energy and all organisms are reliant upon the primary energy transforming action of the plant and algae kingdoms.

The grass and algae, with their magical chlorophyll, assimilate the energy from the sun itself. The gazelle eats the grass and receives the energy of the sun indirectly through it. And the carnivore eats the gazelle to get the sun's energy. But only by eating the entire body and not just a small piece of the muscle, can the carnivore be assured of gaining the entire nutritional value of the sun as received by the grass

Let's switch gears and consider another very apparent, relevant fact: physically, humans are extremely ill-equipped to catch and eat animal prey. Our incisor teeth are nothing like the fang-like canines of carnivores. Imagine trying to kill an animal with your mouth right now. Sure we can invent guns and hunt, but we were not born with guns and arrows. All animals in nature are born equipped for what they need to survive on earth. Our brains are big for sure but just for fun, imagine trying to penetrate the hide of a huge animal with the teeth that you have. Physically, we are not equipped to catch and kill animals.

*We are always free to eat whatever we want whenever we want to! We are also free to have the consequences. Be aware, then do what you want!*

*"There are over fifty thousand different active proteins in the human body, all made out of the same building blocks, amino acids- which, are made of carbon, hydrogen, oxygen, and nitrogen, as well as sulfur, phosphorous, and iron. Some protein molecules are huge and have thousands of amino acids strung together like beads on a necklace."*
*Dr. Jensen's Guide to Body Chemistry*

One more point that is worth making: Psychologically as well, humans are ill equipped to kill and eat animals. Dead and dying animal bodies, with all that blood and guts generally speaking, make most humans a bit squeamish. Do you think a tiger with blood all over his face feels uncomfortable about putting his nose in the still wiggling carcass? Can you imagine putting your nose into a carcass? That is because you were never supposed to. Think about the way those of us who consume flesh do it. The food is far removed from its original source. The animals that carnivores eat are raw and live. No human would eat an animal if it were still alive and very bloody.

Also, when you consider what it means to really eat another mammal, take a moment to consider that the nervous system of a cow or any other mammal reacts the same way as ours when it comes to suffering, terror and the threat of death. All nervous systems signal for the release of adrenaline, cortisone and other highly toxic secretions upon fear of imminent death. All animals have the instinct and the calling towards self-preservation. All animals cherish their lives. To put a creature to death for your food when you should not really be eating it in the first place is silly.

Keep eating fish if you have to. But have no illusions about fish being different. Fish is meat too. There is no good reason to eat fish unless you are literally starving to death, and then the fish better be raw and parasite free. Many foods in the plant kingdom as well as the algae kingdom, have the same essential fatty acids that the fish contain. In fact, the fish that are supposedly beneficial to eat are the algae eaters and that is why they are so high in the beneficial Omega-3 fatty acids. The many different species of Blue-Green Algae form the foundation of the food chain in the oceans. Eating this is valuable for us because their cell walls are made of the same essential fatty acids that our cell walls are made from. Cell walls that are made from good fats like these are flexible and youthful.

Foods like avocado, olives, spirulina and the soon to be introduced 'E-3 Live", contain these Omega-3 Fatty acids of a superior quality.

# Chapter 12- Dairy

Consumption of another animal's milk is bizarre. At your age, is it not difficult to imagine drinking human's breast milk with your breakfast? Is it not stranger to drink the breast milk from some other animal like a cow?

The milk of each species is designed specifically for the young of that species. It is an extremely potent dose of hormones, vitamins, fats and growth factors designed for the offspring's growing body. The rapid body growth and small brain of a calf have different nutritional needs and subsequently, their mothers produce drastically different milk than what our mothers make. Cow's milk contains 300% more casein - the chief protein in milk - than human breast milk. Cows are bovines, a family of hoofed mammals, drastically different from large brained Homo sapiens.

There are a few myths about benefits of eating dairy.[13] That dairy is good for bone density and bone growth is false. This belief comes from the fact that both cow's milk and our bones both contain the mineral calcium. The proposed link of dairy to healthy bone status in women due to its calcium content has led many doctors to recommend dairy consumption. This is unfortunate because dairy is likely the cause of osteoporosis, not the cure.

Though milk does contain calcium, your body must use more calcium than it actually gets from milk in order to process it. When pasteurized milk is digested in your body, the by-products that are left behind are so acidic they actually raise the ph level of the blood. To maintain the precise blood ph level (slightly alkaline) that the body requires, it must neutralize the acidic influence with alkaline substances. Alkaline minerals, mainly calcium, must be leached from the bones where they are stored, and released into the bloodstream to stabilize its ph level. The result is a calcium loss. In short, more calcium is taken out of the bones than put in when one eats dairy.

It has been observed in many studies that osteoporosis is almost non existent in societies where people do not use dairy after infancy. As for dairy and muscle strength, a gorilla does not have a trace of dairy in its diet once it is passed its infantile stage. Yet, a 400 pound gorilla is about thirty times stronger than a 180 pound man.

*One definition of a mammal passing infancy is that it has been weaned. As adult primates we do not need to suckle a bovine.*

*The main ingredient in Elmer's™ glue is casein.*

Another misunderstanding is that only some people are lactose intolerant while others are not. To digest milk, an enzyme called lactase is necessary. It breaks downs the lactose or sugar contained in the milk. In the early stages of a mammal's life, it is equipped with lactase. As it grows, the production of lactase is reduced and the weaning process begins. With less lactase in the system, the offspring suffers cramps when it consumes milk until it eventually refuses to nurse. In adult humans, cow's milk forms large tough curds in the stomach and intestines.

Currently, only the people who suffer extreme discomfort from consuming dairy are labeled 'lactose intolerant' or 'allergic to milk.' Even though we all may not get bloated and experience cramping when we consume dairy, all adults are lactose intolerant to a degree. Less acute symptoms of lactose intolerance are dark circles under the eyes, a runny nose and congestion. If you are familiar with any of these symptoms in your life, you do not have to rely on my word alone, stop consuming dairy for a while and watch how they may disappear.

That we get good protein from dairy is another false assumption. Many experts say that the protein in dairy is not a healthy protein variety for us. In the now famous book <u>The China Study</u>, written about a huge and long term study of nutrition and disease correlations in China, Dr. Campbell explains that there was a direct relationship between protein and cancer saying, "We found that not all proteins had this effect. What protein consistently and strongly promoted cancer? Casein, which makes up 87% of cow's milk protein, promoted all stages of the cancer process. What type of protein did not promote cancer, even at high levels of intake? The safe proteins were from plants."

All lactating (producing milk) mammals must have just given birth or else they would not lactate. If the female cow is giving her milk to a machine for human use then her calf is not getting it. The inevitable result of the human demand for cow's milk is called veal.

## Chapter 13- Water and Non-Water Fluids

Water is so important that it deserves more than a chapter, perhaps an entire book. There is so much to the nature of water that is a mystery and yet taken for granted. Water is the only fluid that is technically a drink; everything else is a 'food'.[14] It is necessary to drink plenty of clean water every day. It is important to drink a large glass of water first thing in the morning to promote peristalsis (bowel movement).

Water is the key ingredient which makes life possible. The human body consists of 70% water as we are essentially miniature oceans walking around earth. Because we must replace our water constantly and drink ample water everyday, the effect of drinking unclean or un-pure water is very serious. Drinking polluted water is a good way to get sick, both short term or long term, depending on the water. Never trust tap water unless you know with **certainty** its quality.

Generally speaking, stay with artesian water because it is usually the result of rain that took place decades ago. Artesian water is any water that rises to the surface as a 'spring' on its own. Artesian water flows upward before emerging. Generally speaking avoid mineral water because the in-organic version of the minerals do little for our bodies except build plaque inside our arteries.[14]

## Soda

Sodas and soft dinks are more like poisons than a drink because they combine high levels of sodium with high levels of refined sugar. With all the food colorings and preservatives, these are pretty toxic. I am not using words like that lightly; that is what they are. Why would we give this to our children?

## Coffee

Coffee is bad mostly for the way caffeine stimulates the adrenal glands to work harder because it is an alkaloid that is recognized as a toxin to be eliminated. The adrenals release more adrenaline after a cup of coffee than is normal. The other problem with coffee, which may be a bigger issue is the sugar, milk or cream that it is

*'Only water cleans!' This is true in your house, and in your body.*

*If possible, avoid Aspartame! It is worse than you can possibly imagine.*

mixed with. Refined sugar is almost the worst thing a person can eat.[16] Aspartame (Nurtrasweet™) is even worse! Cream and milk are dairy.

## Teas and Green Tea

Green tea is probably good for you to some extent but the more caffeine is not the better, generally speaking. English Tea is probably gentler on the body than coffee but the caffeine is still there.

## Juices

Fresh juice is good. Raw fruit sugar- fructose, is the fuel of the brain. Fructose in nature comes with a complete package of fiber, vitamins and enzymes called a piece of fruit. Bottled juices are usually full of refined sugar or heated fruit sugar. These heated sugars are harmful because of the way they deliver a lot of deranged sugar molecules quickly and thus negatively affect blood sugar levels in the body. One reason for this is that there is no nutritional balance to the sugar the way there is in a piece of fruit.

## Alcohol

Alcohol molecules are by their nature anti-life. In fact alcohol molecules kill every living cell they touch. This feeling of the burning down your throat after a 'shot' is the sensation of cells dying after being exposed to alcohol. Even red wine, which is often cited as healthy, is not. The properties of red wine considered healthy are simply found in the grapes. The other major problem with alcohol is how it suppresses everything about our immune system and makes us susceptible and vulnerable in different ways than if we did not have alcohol. Alcohol has some moderate benefits. For example, its tendency for being a social lubricant as well as the benefit of 'relaxation' for the party goers. So drink if you like it and the benefit outweighs the health costs for you but alcohol is highly taxing.

# Section III
## Building a Healthy Foundation

*One way or the other, the body is making one million cells every second, and these cells must be made from something.*

*By allowing more high quality hotistic foods to be consumed, you are planting the seeds, the fruits of which will be reaped as the body's new found strength and will.*

## Chapter 14- Sleep

It would be hard for you to imagine how valuable sleep is to our health. Sleep refuels the liver and cells with glycogen, the fuel that the body uses in the execution of cellular activity. The production of cells is nearly double during sleep so healing and regeneration are much better.

Sleeping is so valuable that it is not possible to oversleep because the rule is that if your body is sleeping, it needs to be. Try to sleep and wake up on your own, without an alarm clock because that means that you have had enough sleep. The body can perform miracles when it is given the full use of its resources and energy.

The best time for sleeping is between 9pm and 5am because these are the hours in the cycle of the day that are most restorative in the human bio-energetic cycles [17]. Try to sleep for as many of those hours as possible. Simply get as much sleep as you can because that is a key to health.

If you do not get all the sleep you need, it is fine to take a nap. The human brain and body love a bit of rest, especially with the stress inducing environment of modern living. The energy regeneration of only 10 minutes of sleep is significant. Lots of healing and restoration takes place in naps. Sleep is the time when the brain regenerates the low-level electricity called nerve energy that is its currency.

Sleep is when the body takes care of itself. If you are ever not feeling well, like you have a 'cold', one way of handling it healthfully is to drink lots of water and sleep until you cannot sleep anymore. One or two 12 to 14 hour night sleeps is the best medicine when we do not feel perfect.

For good sleep, you need: Darkness, Quiet and Coolness. If you don't have darkness, cover your eyes with a shirt or something and have some real darkness. It makes all the difference. Always rest with something covering the eyes if it is not very dark. Fresh air should be allowed in the room.

Meditation is different from sleep. Many claims are made as to the health and rest value of meditation and they are true! Meditation is very restorative in its own right. However, nothing can replace the need for adequate proper sleep.

## Chapter 15- Sunlight

Sunlight is a nutrient for our bodies feeding us a wide spectrum of electromagnetic radiation that our bodies need to absorb. Our bodies need sunlight as opposed to artificial light because the sun offers a powerful and unique energy.

*We need sunlight to make good bones.*

Artificial attempts to imitate sunlight can never be accurate because the sun is a star! We need real sunlight to keep ourselves healthy. Physically speaking, our bone integrity requires the sunlight for Vitamin D production. One of the best things we can do for ourselves is to take a daily sun bath for about 20 minutes. One way to look at it is to see sunlight as a nutrient, along with oxygen, water and food.

The sun is not actually the cause of skin cancer,[18] as strange as that may sound to you. If the sun was the sole cause of skin cancer, humans would not be the only species that gets it. There must be something else! Something 'plus' the excessive sunlight creates the skin cancer. To avoid skin cancer, stop eating refined sugars and pastas and do not stay in the sun for too long at a time.

The sun is the source of life on the planet and the sustainer of our lives. We must have direct exposure to the sun regularly to be healthy. Mentally, sunlight keeps us in balance too. Depression is often associated with a lack of sunlight. There is an important psychological component to the benefits to some direct sun exposure.

We need sunlight to make good bones. The body, when exposed to real sunlight creates Vitamin D[19] which is necessary for the use of Calcium in our bodies. Sunlight, plus resistance based activities like Power Yoga are the key to preventing osteoporosis because they encourage strong bones in two different ways at the same time. Strong bones are created from the inside out, and from the outside in!

Therefore, avoid sunscreen unless absolutely necessary. Sunscreen is an untested (in the longterm) way of blocking certain frequencies of the sun's radiation. A concern with sunscreen is that those formulations contain some very complex molecules that do not need to be rubbed into our skin, which absorbs everything into the bloodstream. If you are ever going to be in the sun for long periods of time, wear long sleeves and a hat instead of poisoning your blood to protect yourself.

## Chapter 16- Silence

"That's my business," "It would be suicide to announce that." [20]

Any one can notice that he who talks too much does not often take action while those who take action seldom talk about it. Consider your body to be a vessel which is a storehouse for energy, as many of the Eastern teachings including Yoga analogize. If the human vessel is releasing its energy through its mouth, then the energy is no longer available to sustain the power and perseverance required for the action.

Talk is cheap and easy and for this reason alone is always suspect when relating to future accomplishments or goals. It is so easy for a person to talk about doing something and so hard for them to actually do it. This may be for a reason that is not so obvious but quite apparent.

The type of person who easily talks about future goals and never realizes them (which is a great percentage of the population) may not realize that it is actually the talking itself which is responsible for the distance between themselves and the subject they are talking about. It is not a coincidence.

Unnecessary talk is often the greatest enemy to the attainment of any goal. As unnecessary talk leaves your mouth, the energy literally drains from your body.

We can observe when we find ourselves talking about what we want to do, and notice how the chance of our actually doing that action diminishes. Then, observe the next opportunity you have to talk about something that is important for you to accomplish but instead, choose not to share it and see how it just gets done.

Wise men and women realize this by speaking only through their actions. Only actions speak. An enlightened person recognizes this by never talking about a situation and only taking action towards its resolution swiftly and directly.

The energy generated during sleep is finite and once expelled is gone until you sleep again. There are many ways which energy can be drained from the body and talk is chief among them. The same energy that goes out of the mouth in words could have been simply put to the task at hand. Stay quiet and keep your power!

## Chapter 17- Drugs, Doctors, and Healing

So often we are told that if we do not feel well we should go to the doctor, and the doctor has to cure the sick body. The assumption is that the body is incapable of taking care of itself. The assumption is also that the body needs to be 'cured' of symptoms. These are both incorrect assumptions.

Firstly, that the embryo and growing baby need no outside assistance to execute perfect development, and that the body always heals itself of cuts on your surface, should make you realize that those innate powers have never left. The same Intelligence is always in you, always striving to bring you to the healthiest version of 'you' possible under the conditions. The intelligence is in every one of the trillions of cells that make up our body. In spiritual language, "You can not separate the Created from the Creator".

But I want to keep impressing upon you that just as the human grows and develops without outside instruction or interference, so too does it heal. Any superficial cut will demonstrate that the body needs no help in the actions of repair. The body is fully self-healing of cuts and scratches is it not?

It was not, for example, necessary to plug the body into a diagnostic machine and download individual commands about where to place particular protein molecules or what order to begin its repair process. These bodily actions are fully self-directed from within the body. This self-direction is what we call Intelligence.

Secondly, generally speaking, symptoms are actions that the body has chosen to express in order to either cleanse itself or tell you something needs to change. Ameliorating the symptom without addressing the cause is not the long term solution.

There is almost no reason to take pharmaceutical drugs and 'over the counter' remedies. Just as we do not need to tell our bodies how to heal a scratch, we need not tell the body how to heal anything. It should not be that hard to believe that the same intelligence that brought you from the embryo to where you are now, has the information it needs to heal itself and put things according to plan. What is needed is not to add toxins.

A common assumption exists that drugs have the ability to seek out specific places and cells. This assumption holds that

*"I don't advise anyone who has no symptoms to go to the doctor for a physical examination. For people with symptoms, it's not such a good idea, either. The entire diagnostic procedure- from the moment you enter the office to the moment you leave clutching a prescription or referral appointment- is a seldom useful ritual."*
*Dr. Robert Mendelsohn*

Tuesday, January 10, 2006
CHICAGO- (AP)-

Drugstore shelves are crowded with cough syrups promising speedy, often non-drowsy relief without a prescription.

But "the best studies that we have to date would suggest there's not a lot of justification for using these medications because they haven't been shown to work," said Dr. Richard Irwin, a professor of medicine at the University of Massachusetts Medical School in Worcester, Mass.

drugs and medications act with intelligence, able to search for and affect certain cells and leave others alone.

Yet, drugs are not endowed with this sort of intelligence. Drugs are just chemical compounds without life-force and without self-direction.

The body is fully self healing within its entire vital domain. The only thing that interferes with that healing process is poisons and poisonous energy patterns. This should be pretty common sense. I hope that it is. The body is the conscious being here, not the doctor's mind. Leave all healing to the body, except in the cases of gunshot wounds, broken bones and the like.

The principles of health are clear. Nothing that makes a healthy person sick can ever make a sick person healthy.[21] A healthy lifestyle, not a chemical, is the solution to imbalance. Only the body heals. The body possesses the intelligence, not the chemical. It does so in the same magical mystical way that you developed in the womb.

Mainstream medicine is not interested in healing people, only in managing for profit their illnesses. One look at most hospitals' menu betrays their intentions. These are managers of human disease and are not experts in human health.

This point is relevant because if we get sick and go to a doctor, we assume that we are going to a human expert. A doctor should be a human expert like a tiger specialist at the zoo is a tiger expert. If a person gets sick, the doctor should be able to know what the requisites are for health in humans, ask the right questions and determine the **cause** of the symptom or disease.

If a tiger specialist learned that a constipated tiger was eating a large deep dish pizza every day, the tiger would be taken off the deep dish pizzas **first**. All other questions would be reserved until after the tiger was put back on its scientifically correct diet. Only after the most logical possible cause has been addressed can more remote possible factors be taken into account.
Why don't our doctors take the same approach? Why don't our doctors ask themselves if what we have eaten is related to what we are feeling? The reason is that, unbelievably, they are not trained in the connection between diet and disease like any proper animal expert would have been.

*"Physician: First, do no harm." Hippocratic Oath*

## Chapter 18- Obstacles Revealed

It is said that our minds are either our best friend or our worst enemy. Our mind is our enemy when it puts obstacles in our path. The obstacles to enlightenment and success are: resistance, negative attitude, guilt and impatience. But obstacles only slow down the traveler when he is unaware of them. Only unseen or unknown obstacles threaten the journey. With awareness you shine a light on these obstacles and you can then step around. As they emerge in your thoughts, simply let them go because with your awareness of their mechanisms, their power is gone.

## Resistance

Here is an example of resistance and non-resistance in our lives: Consider a song which is playing on the radio as you walk in a room that you find rough and a little grating. Since the song is initially disliked you begin to resist it and wish that it would end. This resistance to the song is expressed in a resistance pattern or tension in the body as well. All of a sudden, you realize that the voice of the singer sounds a bit familiar and you recognize it to be your favorite artist. In fact, you were listening to a brand new song by your favorite singer. Instantly, upon this realization, your disposition toward the song changes. You soon feel yourself accepting the music deep into your body and receiving the song with gratitude. Soon you are gently swaying to the music and happy to be listening to the song which is by now recognized to be quite good.

*When we resist in our lives, we hold our breath and become uncomfortable.*

In resistant mode we build walls, feel nervous and irritated, and convince ourselves that we were not happy because of the situation. In the realized mode, we have relaxed the walls and the nervousness subsides and is replaced by a feeling of indescribable wellbeing, connectedness and gratitude.

## Negativity

Our thoughts so profoundly affect our health that it is more dangerous to think negatively than it is to eat negatively or other destructive activities. Negative thought energy may be the most

*Always save your energy wherever you can.    Nuerons require a lot of energy to 'fire'.  Save this energy by letting go of all self-attacking thoughts.*

destructive force endured by our bodies.  All thoughts of guilt, judgment or hate send a barrage of powerful and destructive biochemicals throughout the body.  Because our minds and bodies are 'not two', we can instead positively affect our physical health with a mental attitude that never sends negativiy toward ourselves.  Likewise, we affect our mental and psychological health through good exercise.

## Guilt

Guilt is an expression of negativity where you attack yourself with your thoughts for something that happened in the past.  This self-attack is vicious because there is no defense against it.  The less conscious person is at the mercy of his attacking mind, when a better use of the mind would have been to learn a lesson from the situation and then forgive oneself completely and totally.  Instead of the mind being the ally who is steeped in gratitude, reverence and awareness, the mind becomes the enemy by attacking with the weapon of guilty feelings.  As if guilt could accomplish anything anyway!   Instead of guilt, what is needed is **resolve**. Resolve to never make that mistake again!

Guilt can never accomplish something because it is so draining!  That is why it is never productive to feel guilty. Feeling guilty is always a waste of your limited vital energy.  Punishing yourself for anything done in the past is never appropriate because there is nothing gained and nothing learned.  Past mistakes do hold some value as lessons when future decisions can be made more wisely.  The way to let go of guilty thoughts and other destructive type thoughts is mid sentence!  Let them go mid-sentence and be free.

## Negative Attitude

Since the attitude determines the outcome, a negative attitude creates failure and a positive attitude creates success.  Even if a task is possible, a person with a negative attitude may not accomplish it. On the contrary, a task that seems almost impossible will be easily attained by someone with a positive attitude. The person with a positive attitude is grounded in the knowledge that practice is behind success.

A person with a positive attitude does not say that someone else is **better** at something than him, rather that the person has practiced more. People who are proficient at something have had a lot of practice, a lot of training.

Even those with great natural talent must work and practice tirelessly. Simply, practice is the only means to accomplishing anything or learning how to do anything well. To the person who thinks thoughts with a positive view point, it is not a question of, if a skill will get learned; it is only a question of when! Let your attitude be your means to do anything you want!

## Impatience

Many people are thwarted from success at their undertakings because of unrealistic expectations and impatience. Impatience is the father of frustration. Frustrated due to their false expectations, many beginners give up.

There is so much wasted energy looking at the ultimate goal. The ultimate goal is important as a vision, but then the only way to get there becomes the very next step possible from your present location. In fact, where you actually need to go is the closest place to where you are right now that leads you in the direction of choice.

Very few valuable changes can happen overnight! Expressions like "Nothing easy is ever worth having," and "Patience Pays," have evolved to instruct us. Being like the tortoise and not the hare allows us to arrive at our destination! One way of making patience more practical is in realizing that only the next step matters.

*It is very difficult to stop a person with a positive attitude from accomplishing his goal.*

*No reason to hurry to be somewhere or someone else. Relax, take your time and enjoy the holistic path. How can there be a hurry when you have already arrived?*

One step at a time and moving slowly does the tortoise cross the finish line. Visualize this: if you are going somewhere and you do not take the next, closest step from wherever you are presently, it is not possible to arrive. Only the next step matters because without it movement does not take place in the preferred direction.

Patience may be seen as an ability to accomplish future goals by working diligently on their realization in the present moment. Working in the present moment is the same as *taking the next step*. A truly patient person may even do things that appear not even related to the goal, all the while visualizing how their present actions are the foundation.

# Section IV
## Transformation

*Yoga and eating more raw foods are two of the holistic practices that when incorporated into your life to any degree will immediately and positively affect your life.*

*The transitioning person must make sure his meals are satisfying.*

## Chapter 19- Transition

The first months of a transition time might have no food changes at all and may simply involve the physical practice of Yoga. This will build initial strength and energy reserves, as the exercise invigorates your body and allows you to sleep better.

My philosophy is that for the first several years of transition it is important to make use of rich gourmet raw food selections and avocados. The emotionally satisfying aspect of eating lies in something called satiation, which means feeling full. The feeling of being full and satiated and that of being satisfied are connected. What is needed in a meal is to feel satisfied and full after we are done eating. The transitioning person must make sure his meals are satisfying.

Luckily, there is an entire world of raw foods which is classified *gourmet* and many pleasing and emotionally satisfying foods that are raw. In addition, there is the Avocado. The Avocado may be the most important food for human beings because it provides satisfaction and fullness in a healthful way. The key to transitioning is to stay full. Keep eating as much good food as you can so you are never hungry. When supported by a full belly, a person is not likely to be tempted.

The best way to transition is to evaluate, like a researcher, the effects of foods on your overall feeling and vitality. Without judgment observe with great detail what you eat and then in very great detail, observe both your bowel movement regularity and your level of nasal congestion. Be sensitive to the functioning of the body in a way that you have not before. Then slowly and over a chosen course of time, begin to experiment with eating an entire day of raw foods. Just one day, eat only as much raw food as you want and then go to sleep. Then like a scientist, just evaluate the differences.

If this process takes 2 years, that is great. It takes a long time to make real change and real change only happens when you take things nice and slow. Carefully construct your foundation over a long time. Remember that while the foundation of a building is never seen, it is THE most important part. Just always do the Yoga! Exercise assures the most efficient elimination of the poisons releasing into your bloodstream as the body ejects them in the cleansing process. Also if possible avoid *anti-perspirants* that contain any form of aluminum, which is a toxic metal.

# Chapter 20- Practical Implementation

Here is the best way I have found to approach the practical implementation of the raw foods and Yoga aspects of this path: gently. When you have decided that you want to eat better, you have to practice first!

When you are ready to start practicing eating all raw, you do so for only one day at first. One day eat well, and then go back to your normal food. Next time, maybe a week or two later, do two days. Next time, maybe two weeks later, do three days. Each time return back to your normal food without regard. Just practice. In this way you're flexing the muscles of your will power and developing the mental strength you will need if you want to go for a week or a month 'raw'.

Also try not to get caught answering the 'Are you ever going to eat cooked food again?' question. If you are asked, the best answer is to smile and say 'I don't generally talk about the distant future, only what is likely take to place for the next meal.'

Changing one's diet begins, as explained above, with recognition of the correct meaning of food. As with the Yoga Asanas, the practical implementation involves starting very slowly and working up to increased levels of strength and endurance and flexibility over time, without ever hurrying or applying force. Simply eating more fruits and other high-quality non animal based foods is the most important thing we can do in the early phases because this lays the cellular foundation for exhibiting degrees of discipline and strength previously unimaginable.

Most importantly, with regards to the practical implementation of this knowledge, is how raw foods and Power Yoga support each other and create a positive symbiosis known as a Positive Feedback Cycle. Through time, the feedback cycle results in each aspect getting stronger from the other. It is magical and transformational. Here is how it works:

Let's say you start doing a few 'Sun Salutaions' a day. As you move blood through your body, you oxygenate your tissues. Your blood also becomes cleaner. Day by day, you become more invigorated and a longer more physical practice starts to build strength. As you start to feel stronger and healthier, you become better attuned to your body and you begin to become more conscious of your diet. Through a more regular Yoga practice you start to become aware of how different foods make you feel and

*Never feel like you are being strict with yourself. Everything you do is an experiment, and an opportunity.*

Through a more regular Yoga practice you start to become aware of how different foods make you perform.

perform. Gradually, cravings for the more toxic foods begin to fade. Energized with a healthier diet, you begin to approach your Yoga practice with vigor and intensity, moving through poses that seemed impossible a few months ago. This in turn, strengthens your motivation to eat well.[22]  Soon, eating the real garbage food seems unlikely and going a day without doing your Yoga practice would be like going a day without brushing your teeth. And so on!

With the Positive Feedback Cycle on your side, the practical implementation of this Path is simply a matter of taking your time and enjoying the process. Remember always about the journey being the destination. Have Fun!

## Chapter 21- Sadhana

Another way to consider the practical implementation stuff is in a spiritual light. Make these practices your Sadhana. Sadhana is a Sanskrit word and it means spiritual discipline. Sadhana is whatever spiritual practice the person does daily. Practicing Power Yoga everyday is a Sadhana. My appreciation of the word Sadhana is that because there is a spiritual element, there are no exceptions, no 'days off'.

This is part of my Sadhana: Unless something unforeseeable happens, I am going to do my Power Yoga practice everyday. Some days I will have 25 minutes. Other days I will have 1 hour 25 minutes but everyday without exception I step to my mat and exercise my body as a way of expressing gratitude.

Sadhana is both daily and spiritual and that is why it is so effective. It adds a dimension to which we normally do not access called spiritual power and we continue doing our exercises no matter what. It is a linking of spirituality and discipline. In a way, Sadhana is the train. You get on board and disciplines spill over into each other. The disciplined person can be very powerful. Here is a good example:

Deepak Chopra, one of the most respected health and medical experts in the world, is a powerful Yogi. He begins each day at 4am with Sitting Meditation and Yoga until 6am and then he writes for 2 hours all the material for his many books, and then does some exercise, ALL BEFORE 9AM. He says that he has taken care of his entire being- Mind, Body, Spirit and Livelihood, all before 9am so that everything that happens in the rest of the day is just extra. This is a Sadhana from one of the world's most successful persons not to mention someone who is already maybe the world's greatest healer and doctor.

Anybody can have a Sadhana and it does not have to start out as almost all Raw and practicing yoga 2 hours everyday. Actually it is best if started slowly. Just start by eating one piece of fruit a day more than you would have eaten or start with a bit of Downward Dog everyday.

This is a Sadhana that would take about 1 minute and a half. Yet it is as spiritually powerful as any other. In a few months, taking it very slowly, you can evolve your Sadhana so that you only eat fruit before noon and do 30 minutes of Yoga daily. This is

*It takes 40 days for your new practice to be a Sadhana. It is said that 40 days makes Sadhana.*

*By getting your muscles stronger every day, your will power gets stronger over time.*

powerful stuff and all you have to do is start.

And by the way, whatever happens with your food selections, just keep practicing Power Yoga and everything will unfold in time. Always do the Power Yoga!

## Chapter 22- A Kitchen Set-up

Here are the specifics of the raw kitchen set up. The things you are going to need and the things you may let go of. Take it slow; you do not have to turn into 'the perfect eater' in a week or a month. For those who are ready, these are the instructions to prepare your kitchen.

First of all, if you have not already, throw away your microwave oven. That was a bad invention to begin with and there is no reason to ever use one or be near one when it is operating.

Throw away your table salt and refined sugar. They are poisons and throwing them away is fine. Search for all things in your cupboard with refined sugar, which may use the names: sugar, brown sugar, corn-syrup, high-fructose corn syrup, etc; and artificial sweeteners under the names of NutraSweet™, Aspartame, Splenda™ etc. Aspartame is NutraSweet™ and is a particularly nasty chemical.

Clean your refrigerator of meat and other animal type foods and clean your fridge real good. Throw away stuff when you are sure you are not going to want to eat it. Not because you want to force yourself not to eat it, but because you just feel that it is unlikely that you are going to eat it.

Buy some baskets so you can have fruit and avocadoes ripening in your kitchen. Baskets are great because they are soft enough and can be lifted off the counter or the floor and kept away from the bugs. Avocadoes should be bought early and ripened at home so you know it will not be bruised or damaged. Buy some big glass jars so you can store nuts or seeds in an airtight container.

It is always better to eat organic food whenever given the choice. Organic fruits and vegetables tend to have more vitamins and life-force than their conventionally grown counterparts. But it is always better to eat conventionally grown raw food (washed well) than cooked organic food (which is not food).

Always have lots of food on hand including snack food and fruit and filling, fatty type possibilities so that you are not hungry ever. Fruit, vegetables and almond butter should be stored in the refrigerator. In the cupboards you can keep the Raw Tahini, Raw Nut Butters (new), good salt, Olive Oil and whatever is Raw and does not have to be refrigerated.

*Throw away your microwave.*

*The texture of crunching is often the addictive part, not the potato chip. (In England they are called 'crisps'.)*

Recognize and anticipate your needs and make sure you have the raw alternatives. For example I used to be so addicted to potato chips that I used to not be able to eat any meal without some sort of potato chip with the meal. I needed that crunch. Turns out that the crunch was really all that I needed! Now I use a flax cracker for the same purpose of texture for my meals and it satisfies me the same way. I did not deprive myself of my need for the chip, I just found the "chip" that was food.

      If you have organic farms in your local area, then you are VERY lucky. Support them fully and gladly pay their slightly higher prices. The following is a list of appliances that are very helpful when eating more raw food.

## 'Tools of the Trade':

### Dehydrators:
A great many of the raw recipes that have a cooked or crunchy texture to them use something called a dehydrator. It is essentially a mini oven and a fan only so that the space inside does not exceed 120 degrees Farenheit, which is the highest temperature enzymes can endure without fracturing. Often recipes go in to a dehydrator for 12 hours or so.

### Food processor:
This chops food up really fine or allows you to chop food up to the degree you want. For many recipes, food processors are used to chop nuts or herbs into a size that is usable for the recipe. These are in-expensive appliances that are very useful and allow you to make lots of different types of Raw Food.

### Blender:
Blenders are really good for making smoothies and fruit drinks. You can make a very satisfying fruit smoothie every morning if you have one of these.

## Chapter 23- Potent Allies

Extra-ordinary circumstances call for extra-ordinary measures. We are living a lifestyle and have all grown up eating foods that are so far from ideal that it has created a need for these special allies in the quest toward health and balance. While the following may not have been necessary when humans lived a more natural life, they are now. If any of these subjects appear far out and incredible, study them yourself! These are highly potent allies.

## Electromagnetic Field Protection

Electromagnetic Fields- All cell phones, radios, satellites, computer screens, airplanes and everything 'electronic', function by emitting either surges or streams of electrons. This is something called Electromagnetic Radiation, and the area within the reach of this radiation is termed the Electromagnetic Field.    Cell phones, for example,  are constantly emitting and receiving from satellites these 'signals' even when they are not being used.    Otherwise, how could they ring! These frequencies are termed 'dissonant' frequencies because they disturb the delicate electro-magnetic balance of living cells.

*Maybe this is a hard concept for people to visualize, but they should not leave this particular subject until they do.*

This radiation 'exposure' is a great experiment in our time and we are the lab rats this time because this kind of radiation has only been around since the late seventies, and the amount of devices emitting it has only 'surged' in the late nineties! So we do not know what it is doing for sure but we do know this:  there is an unprecedented exposure to the chaotic pulsations/radiations of these devices in the form of electrons that are bombarding us. This is no small matter because as living beings we are based on a bio-electrical foundation that is easily disturbed.

Thus, certain companies have created pendants and other devices that are designed to help the body protect itself from these harmful/dissonant frequencies. Most function by helping the body resonate more to the earth's protective/harmonic electromagnetic field. I wear two of these necklaces and do not search for the 'proof' that they work. I know that scientifically speaking, it is extremely logical to take this precaution. (earthcalm.com)

*Enzymes are taken as an addition so as to not have to draw upon that 'Bank Account', as well as to help the body digest all of the tiny debris that has built up in the intestinal canal.*

The following are the helpful **additions** that I use in my life everyday. I am including them because they make a remarkable difference! Try this stuff out if you want to evolve your health in a better direction. Period!

## AFA/E3 Live

The best of all the **additions** is something called AFA- Aphanozeminon Flos-Aqua (Latin for 'invisible flower of the water'). This species of Blue-Green algae is a relative of Spirulina but is much more suitable for humans as far as nutritional assimilation and benefits. These are single cell algae that existed billions of years before the development of either plants or animals!

'E3 Live' is a trade name for the only company, presently, that is harvesting and delivering the AFA in its frozen, vitally intact form. It is a whole, wild, live food and because of some astounding properties this is the only recommendation that, no matter who you are or what your health situation is, you will feel the difference! Personally speaking, 'E3 Live' has done more to improve my strength than anything else with the muscle power that it creates being utterly impressive. Maybe it is because it is the highest known source of protein on earth and in particular has more real Vitamin B-12 than anything else on earth. I eat 'E3 Live' daily and get all my Vitamin B-12 through that. In general Vitamin B-12 deficiency is not common and in almost all cases, is found in meat-eaters not vegetarians. 'E3 Live' is beneficial for all mammals including your pets. (E3live.com)

## Enzymes

Enzymes are a kind of protein that usually have a metallic or active aspect. The active aspect, often based on zinc or other trace metal, is literally the spark of life because of the stored energy in the metal itself. It is the catalyst for all bio-chemical activity in the body.

We are all born with an 'Enzyme Bank Account'. This is a hefty supply of internally based enzymes which is  animating the trillions of bio-chemical reactions happening every day.  While we are born with this intrinsic supply, it is beneficial to add enzymes into your system.  These added enzymes  clear the intestines and gastro-intestinal tract.  In addition to that,  the correct enzymes, once finished digesting and clearing the gastro-intestinal tract, will then travel into the blood vessels where they hydrolyze (decompose) the arterial plaque.  This is a way of regaining the elasticity of your blood vessels, which is one marker of youth. [23]

*The benefits of these allies are beyond my ability to describe.*

Eating cooked food is so draining on us because when the enzyme content is damaged in the heat, it requires us to draw enzymes from our internal reserves to process it.  Over the long-term, this leads to the exhaustion of our reserves.  Eating enzymes as an "addition" is one way to begin to reverse the trend. (E3live.com)

## Probiotics

In a healthy human digestive tract, there are over 40 species of synergistic bacteria/micro-organisms.  These different species are responsible for producing various compounds that our bodies do not produce as well or at all.  They have their jobs to do and for their service, we provide them with a warm body to live in.  They are supposed to be there!

When they are 'home' and 'manning their posts', there is less chance that an unfriendly bacteria can find any 'soil' to grow in. The pro-biotic addition literally plants the seeds of species found in the healthy human gastrointestinal tract. Anybody who has taken antibiotics or drinks a lot of alcohol, has wiped out their stock of healthy bacteria.  (E3live.com)

## Whole Salt

Our cells are bathed in a solution of water and salt at all times.  The bonds of salt are electric and  this electric energy is released only when salt is mixed with water![24]

Where table salt is a refined product, whole salt is a food that feeds the body deeply by supplying trace minerals and electrolytes (electrically charged minerals).

Table salt is an aggressive molecule made up only of the elements Sodium and Chlorine. Instead of containing everything in the periodic table of elements and minerals, table salt only contains sodium and chlorine. It is thus, a highly imbalanced creation that is dangerous inside our body and because of the fact that it is a salt, dissolves and affects the blood easily. Himalayan crystal salt is a whole salt extracted by hand and is perfect for recipes and anything else 'salt' is used for. Table salt should be thrown away. Sea salt is not as bad as table salt but the best salt is 'Himalayan Crystal Salt', from the Hunza region of the Pakistani Himalayas. (americanbluegreen.com)

## MSM (MethylSulfonyMethane)

*Check out the MSM! Your body uses organic sulfur in many important ways including in the make-up of your most powerful anti-oxidants.*

The S in the MSM stands for Sulfur. One of the properties of sulfur is its special ability to neutralize dangerous chemicals and molecules. The Sulfur atom is the active 'site' of many of our most important anti-oxidants like Superoxide Dismutase. Sulfur is also particularly useful to have in the body to provide for rebuilding and healing all kinds of tissue. I get MSM from a product called *Renew Me*, made by the company that harvests the 'E-3 Live.' (E3live. com)

## Lara Bars

These are 100% raw bars that I love because they are in the packaging that allows them to stay fresh without refrigeration. You can find them at your local health food store. If not, be pro-active and have the manager order them! (larabar.com)

There are also catering ser-
vices and many restaurants
emeging all over the United States that are aware of
holistic raw foods.

In New York City there is
Quintessence and Bonobos
restaurants.

In Los Angeles there is the
famous Juliano's, and on
South Beach (Miami) there
is Afterglow.

## Appendix A- Recipes

It is amazing how gourmet and delicious raw foods can be! If you like to be in the kitchen, the things you can create are really diverse and satisfying on all levels. If you have never tried Raw Food recipes, then it is necessary for you to just go out and try them. They are beyond what you would have perceived possible in terms of taste, texture, and satisfaction. Also, besides the following recipes, many great recipe books are available to assist you in the transition towards more raw foods in your diet. For example, Sunfood Cuisine by Frederick Patentoude is excellent!

C=cup/ t=teaspoon/ T=tablespoon

## Deserts:

MANGO PUDDING

2 Mangos
Shredded Coconut & Chopped Pecans, to taste

Use a vegetable peeler to peel mangos. Then place a knife flush to one of the flat sides of the mango pit and cut the mango away from the pit. Add lime if desired and blend until perfectly smooth.

To complete the dessert, pour into dessert cups/dishes and add shredded coconut and chopped pecans or walnuts to taste.


STRAWBERRY CREAM

Half Cup soaked Almonds
2-3 cups Strawberries
1-2 Bananas

Mix soaked almond together with 1.5 cups of Strawberries and 1-2 Bananas. Try not to add any Water (only add if necessary). Mix everything until it gets very creamy. It's delicious!

BROWNIES

Ingredient list:
3 Cups Flax meal
1 1/2 Cups raw Carob powder
4 Cups Raisins
1 T Almond butter

Blend in Food Processor until mixed thoroughly. Press onto flat
non-stick surface and roll out evenly with a baker's roller. Serve.
Can be kept fresh, covered and refrigerated for up to two weeks.
Let stand out of fridge for one hour before serving.


CHOCOLATY CREAM PIE

Ingredient List for Filling:
3 Cups Avocado
14-16 Dates
1 T Olive Oil
1 1/2 T Pumpkin seed butter
1/2 cup raw Carob powder.
1 Cup Water
Ingredient List for Crust:
4 Cups raw Pecans
1/2 cup raw Carob powder
2 1/2 cups Raisins.

Make the crust first by combining all ingredients into Food Processor and pulse thoroughly until blended. Place mixture in Pie Dish and press firmly along sides until crust is formed.

For the Filling, combine all the ingredients into Food Processor until blended. Pour filling into crust and chill for 1-2 hours in fridge or until firm.

BASIC CHEESECAKE

Ingredient List:
6 Cups soaked Almonds
3 T Lemon Juice
2 T Vanilla

Place ingredients into Food Processor and slowly add Water until mixture is smooth and thick. Pour into 10" cake ring and let set for 4 hours in fridge or until firm. Once firm, top with favorite fruit spread (directions below) and let set for another hour. Remove ring binder and serve.

Fruit topping: In Food Processor, combine 1 Cup favorite Berries, 1/2 cup Raisins, 1/4 cup Water. Blend and run mixture through fine mesh sieve.

## Salad Dressings and Sauces:

CARROT GINGER SALAD DRESSING
In a blender, 3 Large Carrots, 1 large thumb Ginger, 1 cup organic Raisins, 1 T Himalayan Crystal salt, 1 T Garlic powder, 1 teaspoon Black Pepper, 2 C Water, 1 C Olive oil.
4 cups dressing made.

## CAESAR SALAD DRESSING

In a blender, 2 Avocados, 8 Dates, 2 T Garlic powder, 2 T salt, 1 T Black pepper, 1 T Dulse powder, 1 t Mustard powder, 1/2 C dried Coconut, 1 C apple cider Vinegar, 2 C Water, 1 C Olive oil. 5 Cups yield.

## MARINARA SAUCE

Ingredients:
4 cups soaked Sun dried tomatoes and 4 cups of soak water.
8 dates
2 T Basil
2 T Oregano
2 T Dried Parsley
2 T Garlic powder
1/2 Onion
1 T whole Salt
1 T Black Pepper
1/4 cup Olive oil

In a blender, place the Sun-dried Tomatoes (re-hydrated) and soak water and all other ingredients. Blend slowly adding water until thickness desired.

## AVOCADO MAYO

In a blender, mix the following, 3 Avocados, 10 Dates, 2 T Salt, 2 T Garlic powder, 1 T Mustard Powder, 1 t Black Pepper, 1 cup apple cider Vinegar, 1 C Water, 1 C Olive oil. Blend until smooth.

# Breads, Lunches and Dinners

## SESAME FLAX BREAD

Tools: Food Processor, Dehydrator with Teflex Sheets (Excalibur™ Dehydrator Recommended)

Pour onto Teflex sheet over the dehydrator rack, smooth out with a spoon, dehydrate 8-12 hours and turn over the flax on the other side removing Teflex sheet to do so.  Dehydrate 4 hours.

ITALIAN TOMATO FLAX BREAD

2T Fennel seeds, 1 C  Rehydrated Sun-Dried tomatoes and soak water, 1T Garlic Powder, 1T Salt, 1T Pepper, 2T Italian seasoning.  Blend until pureed, add 4 C flax meal or seeds, add water while blending.

SUSHI ROLLS

Make as many as desired!  Quantity of your choice!
Sheets seaweed (nori - dried not roasted)
grated Carrot
Avocado
Cucumber
Nama shoyu (un-pastuerized soy sauce)
Slice Cucumber in thin lengths and
lie on Seaweed  then put grated Carrot;
use quarter Avocado then slice in half,
lie next to Cucumber, sprinkle with
Tamari and roll up.

NO-CHICKEN-SALAD

Ingredient List:
5 Cups Soaked Walnuts
1 large Onion
2 large Carrots
1 large Bell Pepper
1 stalk Celery
1/4 cup Olive Oil
1 T Salt
2 T Poultry Seasonings
3 Cups Avocado Mayo (see above for description)

Directions: In a Food Processor, pulse one at a time and place each one in a large bowl after it has been pulsed- carrots, onion, bell pepper, celery, and walnuts.  Add to the bowl the olive oil, salt, seasonings and avocado mayo and mix all ingredients.
Yields 10 Cups.


ALMOND RICOTTA (For Pizzas and Lasagna!)

Ingredients:
6 Cups soaked Almonds
2 Cups dry Coconut
6 sprigs of fresh Rosemary (stripped)
Juice of 2 large Lemons
1 Cup Olive Oil
2 Cups Water
1 T Salt
1/2 T Black Pepper

Directions:  In a Food Processor put the Almonds, Coconut, Rosemary, Lemon juice, Salt and Pepper and blend together. Scrape the sides, then add  slowly while blending the Olive oil and Water.  If too much water, add shredded coconut. Chill one hour before serving.

Yields 10 cups


MOCK TUNA

4 C walnuts soaked overnight in 8 Cups water, strained.
Pulse in food processor until chunky, then place in large bowl.
4 stalks celery pulsed until chopped finely and add to bowl.
1 Red Onion
1/4 cup Dulse (a seaweed)
2 C Avocado Mayo
Mix by hand

ITALIAN WALNUT BALLS

Ingredients:
5 Cups soaked Walnuts
6-8 pitted Dates
1⁄4 cup Olive oil
1⁄4 cup Water
1 T Garlic powder
3 T Fennel seed
2 T Dried Oregano
2 T dry Basil
2 T dried Parsley
1 Red Bell Pepper
2 T Paprika
1⁄4 cup Nama Shoyo
1 T whole Salt
1 T Black Pepper

Soak Walnuts in 10 Cups water for 8-10 hours. Strain and place in food processor.
Add 6 Dates, 1 cup Olive oil, 2 T Garlic powder, 2 T Fennel seeds, 2 T Italian seasonings,
1 T Paprika, 2 T Nama Shoyu. 1T Salt, 1 T Black Pepper, 1 T Cayenne and blend adding water slowly until smooth and thick.
Scoop small Ball-shapes onto de-hydrator sheets and de-hydrate for 12 hours.

FRED'S 'FAMOUS' SALAD

My staple meal is a salad that is simply romaine lettuce mixed with a dressing made from Raw Tahini, Water, Himalayan Salt, and Lemon Juice. The dressing is made first by mixing equal parts of Tahini to Water and Lemon juice, and then add the Salt, and mix it all up until it emulsifies and turns a lighter color and is uniform in texture. Then, I just add the lettuce into the bowl and I can be eating 7 minutes after I walk in the door. No matter how hungry I am, this meal satisfies me, especially when I have my Flax crackers by my side. Maybe you can eat this as often as me, maybe not but you at least have this really quick and satisfying option at your disposal.

## ALMOND PATE

Ingredient List:
6 Cups soaked Slmonds
1 bunch Cilantro
1 bunch Parsley
3 Big sprigs fresh Dill or T of dry Dill
2 T dry Oregano or Basil
1/4 cup Lemon Juice
1/2 teaspoon Mustard Powder
2/3 cup of Olive oil
1 3/4   cups of Water
Dash of Cayenne
T of Salt, Pepper.

Start in a processor:  1 bunch Cilantro, 1 bunch Parsley, 3 sprigs
Dill, 2 T dry oregano or basil (optional), 1 T salt, 1 T black pepper,
dash Cayenne, 1/2 t Mustard powder, 1/4 cup Lemon juice, 1/4 cup
water.Blend one minute, and stop.  Add: 6 Cups soaked almonds,
blend one minute, scrape sides, turn on processor and while it is
running add 1 1/2 cups water, and 2/3 cup Olive oil.
Blend until smooth.
Best if chilled one hour before serving.

## ALMOND –CURRY PATE

Ingredients:
6 Cups oaked Almonds
1 Cup dry Coconut
8 Dates (pitted) or Figs
3/4 cup Olive oil
2 cups Water
1 T whole Salt
1 T Garlic powder
3 T Curry powder

Directions: In processor, take the Almonds, Coconut, Dates, Salt, Pepper, Garlic Powder and Curry Powder and blend for 30 seconds. Then slowly add the water and olive oil while still blending until the consistency is correct for you.

## CORN CAKES

Ingredient List:
5 Cups Almonds
4 T Oregano
4 T Cumin
Dash Cayenne
2 T Paprika
2 T Garlic Powder
2 T Salt
1 1⁄2 Cups Water
1⁄2 Cup Olive oil

Place Almonds and all dry ingredients into Food Processor and blend 30 seconds.
Slowly add 1⁄2 Cup oil and 1 1⁄2 Cup water.
When finished spoon 1/3 -1/2 cup of mixture onto dehydrator sheet and flatten with fork to allow proper de-hydration.
Dehydrate 8-12 Hours. Use spatula to remove from tray.

This is a great recipe for parties and guests. You can eat these Corn Cakes with a fresh salsa. They are sure to be a hit with everyone who tastes them.

## VEGGIE BURGERS

1 large red Onion
1 large Bell Pepper
3 Carrots
1 small head Cauliflower
1 lg. stalk Broccoli
1 C Almonds, soaked 12-24 hours
1 C Sunflower seeds, soaked 5-6 hours
1/4 C Sesame seeds, soaked 5-6 hours
5 cloves Garlic
2 T Water mixed with crystal salt
1 t Cumin
2 T dried Cilantro or 1-2 C fresh

Blend all of the above ingredients and seasonings in a champion juicer with solid plate or a food processor. This blended food is your patty mixture. Form and put 1/2" thick patties on a teflex sheet and place trays in dehydrator. Dehydrate at 105 degrees for 8-12 hours or until desired texture is obtained. Flip your burgers after 4 hours and remove teflex sheets. Continue to dehydrate for 4-5 hours or until desired moisture is obtained. Makes 4 burgers.

# Appendix B- The Pottenger Cat Study

The Pottenger Cat Study was done between 1932 and 1942 and was described in full in the book called Pottenger's Cats by Francis M. Pottenger, Jr., M.D. Dr. Pottenger worked with Alvin Foord, M.D., professor of pathology at the University of Southern California and pathologist at Huntington Memorial Hospital in Pasadena. This study met rigorous scientific standards and was done with nine hundred cats, six hundred of which had complete medical histories, and medical observations were recorded on all the cats.

The comparisons between the cooked meat cats and the raw meat cats were fascinating.

The following comes from the summary of "The Pottenger Cat Study" found in the highly recommended book Conscious Eating by Gabriel Cousens.

'The normals were all uniform in size and development without any skeletal, tissue tone, or fur changes. The calcium and phosphorus content of their bones remained consistent, and internal organs showed full development. They were resistant to infections, fleas and parasites and showed no signs of allergies. Their mental states were friendly, with purring and predictable behavior patterns. They maintained a high level of nervous system coordination. They reproduced one homogenous generation after another, all in good health. The mothers had no trouble with the birth process or nursing. The average litter was five kittens, with the average weight being one hundred nineteen grams.

In contrast, cats fed the cooked-meat diet gave birth to heterogeneous offspring with many variations in skeletal structure. By the third generation, their bones became as soft as rubber. All deficient generations of cats suffered heart problems, nearsightedness and farsightedness, under activity or inflammation of the thyroid and bladder, arthritis and inflammation of the joints, inflammation of the nervous system with paralysis and meningitis, and infections of the kidney, bones, liver, testes, and ovaries. There was also a general decrease in the health of the visceral organs.'

*In this study, observe how the cats that ate the cooked meat ended up with the same diseases that humans get.*

*Yoga teachers who are interested in the development of their student's asana and spiritual practice in a real way will want to begin to elucidate the difference between healthy and not so healthy vegetarian eating.*

## Appendix C- Questions and Answer

Yoga teachers usually talk about being vegetarian or vegan, isn't that enough?

It is certainly indicative of a higher state of consciousness to choose to be a vegetarian or vegan. But there are so many examples of sick vegans that it seems to give a bad rap to being vegetarian. Look, you can be vegan and eat lots of white sugar. Vegan can mean beer, vegan is bread and pasta and if you eat lots of this stuff, even if you don't eat meat, you will not be healthy. So it may be a transition to go vegetarian first and this is likely a good idea if you are so inclined. However recognize that cooked vegetarian fare is not really healthy. Obviously it is healthy compared to a hamburger, but Yoga teachers who are interested in the development of their student's asana and spiritual practice in a real way will want to begin to elucidate the difference between healthy and not so healthy vegetarian eating. 75% raw is a great place to start.

What is Cancer?

One understanding is that cancerous cells are those who have a genetic misconstruction so that they do not respond to the body's efforts to make them part of the community. Basically, they are out of control growers. They grow and grow receiving only their own instructions, not the instructions from the overall intelligence of the body. Certain "foods", drug use, alcohol use, environmental toxin exposure, and radiation exposure are all reasons Genetic/DNA formulation can be skewed with the result being a single "cancerous" cell. This mutation of cells is not uncommon and the body has a most formidable series of procedures to neutralize all cells that are not responding as they should. Any and every cell that no longer listens to the community and tries to grow without regard is destroyed by a powerful group of defensive cells known collectively as our "white blood cells".

My view of cancer is that it occurs because before the defective cell is destroyed, it feeds and thus survives. Cancer cells feed on protein molecules. Ultimately they thrive by feeding only on the deranged (cooked) protein molecules which are circulating in the blood and because their food supply never runs out (i.e. the person doesn't change their diet), the cancer cells are difficult to vanquish. The cancerous cell in its first few days of life simply gorges on all the excess protein in the blood of an average eater. It is not the mutation that is the problem because mutation can occur from natural causes also. Rather it is the combination of the mutation with the excess protein, the soil in which the seedling cancer cell can begin to grow. In my opinion, this cancerous growth process can not happen as easily in the body of someone who eats minimal if any animal proteins because there is no soil for the seeds to grow, and the body can get the job done of neutralizing them before they grow out of its control.

Studies on the subject point to a correlation between cancers and animal based protein consumption.[25]  Another link is between cooked fat and cancers. The link "really was the rule more than the exception," said Eugenia Halle, the head researcher of the study.[26]

Whatever the exact cause of a person's cancer, in my opinion, there is only one course of action. Stop feeding it! Stop feeding cancer what it wants to eat: animal proteins. If you have cancer and you want to get rid of it, you probably want to go to a fasting/healing center like Hippocrates Institute in Palm Beach[27], Florida. While that is an oversimplification due to the complexity of many peoples' disease process, I can say for sure that in my view, the best course of action is one of these healing retreat centers that have M.D. supervised fasting as their methodology. If you want to prevent cancer, simply practice what you have learned in this book.

*Aminal protein and cancer are now correlated.*

## Appendix D- God and Nature

*The Divine must be expressed somewhere on this planet. It is expressed in Nature and all Life.*

     Nature is an expression of the Divine. To me, God and Nature are interchangeable words. My favorite means of expressing this idea comes by alluding to a grade school lesson children in America are taught about Native American spiritual and religious beliefs. A "God of Trees", and a "God of Rain" is what we were taught they believed in. Now if we use "as" (a more correct translation) instead of "of", it makes more sense. 'God of the Eagle' becomes 'God as Eagle'. It is an understanding that all living beings and aspects of nature are expressions of the Divine.

     We have a wonderful brain but it is prone to an illusion of separation from nature. It is no wonder that trips out into nature are so recharging for people. When we look at Nature, the silence and presence often elicit spiritual epiphany and growth sometimes without our realizing.

     Almost everyone wishes in some way to connect to nature or wild animals. There is something intrinsic and deep about this urge to connect with wild animals and nature. But the truth is that we can not be separate from nature because as human beings we are nature's most complex and most perfect creation.

# Appendix E- Online Resources

On-line Resources

## miamiyoga.com
Official website of the Miami Yogashala on South Beach, my Yoga academy. This site has links and information on lifestlye and yoga teacher trainings on Miami Beach, and retreats around the world.

## rawfood.com
Nature's First Law is a leader in the worldwide raw food health movement and this site is a great resource to get food and other stuff delivered. David Wolfe's book Eating for Beauty is highly recommended and can be purchased through their site.

## bakingforhealth.com
They ship some great tasting desert and savory raw foods that are excellent for breakfast or traveling.

## larabar.com
The fore-mentioned Lara Bar can also be shipped directly by the company.

## glaserorganicfarms.com
This Miami based company ships all over the world a full line of organic raw foods that can be the foundation of your diet. I eat their food everyday and am so grateful that they are based close by! But they ship so it doesn't matter where you live!

## gopalshealthfoods.com
Raw cookies that are different flavors and are all good. I love these when I travel or keep them in the car because they don't need to be refrigerated.

## lydiasorganics.com
Go to this site and see all the cool raw snacks and foods available.

## americanbluegreen.com
The source for Himalayan Crystal Salt.

## Appendix F- 5-Day Menu

MONDAY

AM
Fruit- At least 3 times your usual serving
Lara Bar-2 or 3 with Almond Butter

Lunch
Salad with Raw Dressing and Pate
Flax Crackers- as many as you want
Fruit for Desert with Lara Bar or Balls from Bakingforhealth.com

Dinner
Pate with Flax Crackers
Salad with Raw Dressing
Raw dessert.


TUESDAY

AM
Granola from Bakingforhealth.com
Fruit- At least 3 times your usual serving
Lara Bar (there are over seven different selections)-2 or 3
Almond Butter

Lunch
Salad with Raw Dressing and Different Pate
Sprouts of your choice
Flax Crackers- as many as you want
Lara Bar or Balls from Bakingforhealth.com

Dinner
Entrée- Raw Pizza
Pate with Flax Crackers
Salad with Raw Dressing
Raw dessert.

WEDNESDAY

AM
Granola from Bakingforhealth.com
Fruit- At least 3 times your usual serving
Lara Bar (there are over seven different selections)-2 or 3
Almond Butter

Lunch
Salad with Raw Dressing and Different Pate
Raw Sandwich on Flax Bread with Avocado
Flax Crackers- as many as you want
Lara Bar or Balls from Bakingforhealth.com

Dinner
Entrée- Raw Nori Rolls-As many as you can eat.
Salad with Raw Dressing
Raw dessert.

THURSDAY

AM
Granola from Bakingforhealth.com
Fruit- At least 3 times your usual serving
Lara Bar(there are over seven different selections)-2 or 3
Almond Butter

Lunch
Salad with Raw Dressing and Different Pate
Guacamole –As much as you want
Flax Crackers- as many as you want
Lara Bar or Balls from Bakingforhealth.com

Dinner
Entrée- Raw Lettuce Wraps-As many as you can eat.
Salad with Raw Dressing
Raw dessert.

FRIDAY

AM
Granola from Bakingforhealth.com
Fruit- At least 3 times your usual serving
Lara Bar (there are over seven different selections)-2 or 3
Almond Butter

Lunch
Fruit first then wait.
Salad with Raw Dressing and Different Pate
Flax Crackers- as many as you want
Lara Bar or Balls from Bakingforhealth.com

Dinner
Entrée- Raw Lasagna
Raw Bread of your choice
Salad with Raw Dressing

# Recommended Reading

Ageless Body, Timeless Mind by Deepak Chopra M.D.
(Harmony Books, New York, New York, 1993)

All Books by Dr. Masaru Emoto

Anatomy of Hatha Yoga by H. David Coulter
(Body and Breath Inc., Honesdale, Pennsylvania, 2001)

Biological Transmutations by C. Louis Kervran
(Happiness Press, Magalia, California, 1998 edition)

Confessions of a Medical Heretic by Robert S. Mendelsohn, M.D.
(Contemporary Books, Chicago, Illinois, 1979)

Conscious Eating by Gabriel Cousens, M.D.,
(North Atlantic Books, Berkeley, California, 2000)

Eating For Beauty by David Wolfe
(Maul Brothers Inc., San Diego, California, 2002)

Living Foods For Optimum Health by Brian R. Clement
(Prima Publishing, Rocklin, California, 1998)

Mucusless Diet Healing System by Arnold Ehret
(Ehret Literature Publishing Company, Yonkers, New York, 1953 edition)

Natural Hygiene- The Pristine Way of Life by Herbert M. Shelton
(American Natural Hygiene Society, Tampa, Florida, 1994 edition)

Power Vs. Force, The Eye of the I, and I by David R. Hawkins, M.D., Ph.D.
(Hay House, Inc., Carlsbad, California)

Power of Now, The by Eckhart Tolle
(New World Library, Novato, California, 2000)

Prophet, The by Kahlil Gibran
(Alfred A. Knopf, New York, New York, 1962 edition)

Sunfood Cuisine by Frederic Patenaude
(Genesis 1:29, San Diego, California, 2002)

Water and Salt-The essence of life by Peter Ferreira
(Natural Resources inc. 2003)

## Notes

1. New York Times 3/9/04

2. New York Times 4/9/04

3.  The Institute of Medicine, the division of the National Academies which issues the official recommendations to the U.S. about health, doubled the amount of exercise they suggest to 1 hour daily. This revised 'Recommendation' was made in late 2002, meaning that the information about exercise most learned in school is now outdated.

4. 'Karma' Yoga is practiced as surrendering the fruits of your actions.  The 'Karma' yogi would do a good deed and not wish recognition for it.  The person who does a good deed only if there is recognition surrounding it, is not doing 'Karma' yoga, only doing a good deed.

5. The 'Jnana' yogi may study the scriptures or use the mind as the vehicle to connecting with the God/Self-realization.

6. 'Sutra' is the word for stitch and implies short and concise connective poetry where all information is given but only to the initiated can it be understood.  In other words, to ensure safety with the information, some of the details were left to be only delivered verbally by the master to those worthy of the power that the information may bring.

7.  There are presently two uses of the Sanskrit word "Ashtanga" which translates to 'Eight Limbs'.  One use of the word implies the specific set of poses of Ashtanga Vinyasa as taught by Sri Pattabhi Jois in Mysore, India.  The same word is used in the more generalized Hatha yoga way to mean the 'Eight Limb Path' of Raja Yoga as set forth by Patanjali.  In essence they are the same.

8. Andrey Lappa <u>Universal Yoga</u>

9 "When the B vitamin, Thiamin, is destroyed by boiling or overcooking, it is not available to work as a coenzyme with four different enzymes that require thiamin before they can break down carbohydrates to produce energy.  What happens then?  The usual series of steps to make energy is broken, and intermediate proteins from the disrupted process build, producing toxic levels in the cells.  Other enzymes and macrophages are diverted from other tasks in the body to detoxify the overload of these useless proteins." <u>Dr. Jensen's Guide to Body Chemistry and Nutrition</u>

10.  Meat gets stuck in the little pockets of the intestines because meat is devoid of fiber.

11. See description of Pottenger Cat study in Appendix.

12. Carbohydrate-Any of a class of organic compounds that can be broken down to release energy in the animal body.

13. Dairy in ancient India was received with gratitude from the Cow that was standing in its yard when he woke in the morning. The milk was raw, fresh and received in a spiritual way leading to the reverence of cows in India for their life giving milk. This is still observed in India today. Milk in the western world is a different substance entirely.

14. I write 'food' in quotes because it is only really a food if it is nourishing. If the fluid is not nourishing, like if it is a soda-pop, then it is not a food or a drink. A fluid like that could reasonably be called a poison or a drug.

15. According to The Shocking Truth About Water by Paul Bragg, mineral water, due to the inorganic minerals (which are like sediment) that it contains, is a contributor to atherosclerosis- the hardening of the arteries.

16. The book Sugar Blues by William Duffy describes the facts about sugar.

17. Bio-rhythms in all mammal species have been observed.

18. The cause of skin cancer is probably sun mixed with refined sugars in the blood and since there is now less protective ozone, moderating your exposure to the sun in the middle of the day is wise.

19. Vitamin D, is not a vitamin in a technical sense but is a misnamed steroid hormone critical in its role of assimilating calcium into the bones.

19. Andrey Lappa Universal Yoga.

20. New York Times 7/29/02. Lance Armstrong was asked in 2002 about how many more Tour de Frances he would attempt to win.

21. Robert Snaidach

22. It is literally the abdominal muscles that create the will power of a person. There exists a vast network of nerve cells in the belly and there is a direct relationship between will power and strength of abdominal musculature.

23. Flexibility is an agent of youth and is a major factor in determining 'biological' age which is different from chronological age.

## Notes

24. <u>Water and Salt-The Essence of Life</u>

25  <u>The China Study</u>- Startling Implications for Diet, Weight Loss, and Long Term Health    T. Colin Campbell, PHD

26 New York Times  4/24/03 In regards to the methodology of this study, Dr. Donna Ryan, head of a Biomedical Research Center in Baton Rouge said, "Because of the magnitude and strength of the study, it's irrefutable."

27.  Founded by Bryan Clemens, this healing center offers Medically Supervised fasting programs that have healed cancer and other diseases.

# Index

# Index

# Index

# Index

# Index

# Index

Printed in the United States
49034LVS00005B/87-132